Guidelines for the Care of
Migrant Farmworkers' Children

This publication was funded through an educational grant from Whole Foods Market.

Guidelines for the Care of Migrant Farmworkers' Children was developed through the cooperative efforts of the American Academy of Pediatrics Committee on Community Health Services and the Migrant Clinicians Network.

The recommendations in this publication do not indicate an exclusive course of treatment or serve as a standard of medical care. The guidelines are general and are intended to be adapted to many different situations, taking into account the needs and resources particular to the child, family, locality, and type of practice. Variations and innovations that improve the quality of patient care are to be encouraged rather than restricted.

Library of Congress Catalog Card No.: 99-80164

ISBN: 1-58110-044-2

MA0150

Inquiries may be directed to

American Academy of Pediatrics
Division of Community Health Services
141 Northwest Point Blvd
PO Box 927
Elk Grove Village, IL 60009-0927

Migrant Clinicians Network
PO Box 164285
Austin, TX 78716

Cover photos: Boy and girl picking berries courtesy of Alan Pogue.

Editor
Jennie McLaurin, MD, MPH, FAAP

Assistant Editor
Carmen Retzlaff, MPH, CHES, *Community Health Education Concepts*

AAP Committee on Community Health Services 1997–1998
Paul Melinkovich, MD, Chairperson
Wyndolyn Bell, MD
Denice Cora-Bramble, MD
Helen Du Plessis, MD, MPH
Stanley I. Fisch, MD
Robert E. Holmberg, Jr, MD
Arthur Lavin, MD
Carolyn J. McKay, MD, MPH
Denia A. Varrasso, MD
David L. Wood, MD, MPH

Contributors
Joaquin Borrego, Jr
Leticia Camacho, JD, MA
Armando Correa, MD, FAAP
Melchor Gámez García
Don Gargas, MD, FAAP
Mary Ellen Good, RN, MS, MPH
Mark Koday, DDS
Phillip Landrigan, MD
Ivette Lopez-Bledsoe, MSW
Jennie McLaurin, MD, MPH, FAAP
Kristine McVea, MD, MPH, FAAP
Mark Miller, MD, FAAP
David Rainey, MD, MPH, FAAP
Frederick Rivara, MD, MPH, FAAP
Karen Gordon-Sosby, MSPH, CHES
Anthony Urquiza, PhD
Suzanna Young, RD, MPH

Agency Liaisons
Thomas F. Tonniges, MD, *American Academy of Pediatrics*
Jillian Hopewell, MPA, MA, *Migrant Clinicians Network*
Laura Aird, MS, *American Academy of Pediatrics*
Ana Garcia, MPA, *American Academy of Pediatrics*

Table of Contents

Foreword vii

Purpose and Use of the Manual ix

Chapter 1: Introduction 1
  Background...1
  Understanding the Cultural Context....................................6
  Bilingual Interpreters in the Clinical Setting 28
  Educational Structures in Countries of Origin 34
  Resources 38

Chapter 2: Health Care Guidelines 43
  Well-Child Visits..43
  School Readiness 51
  Immunizations 55
  Adolescent Care 62
  Oral Health 67
  Nutritional Status 76
  Environmental Concerns 83
  Child Maltreatment..96
  Injuries 99
  Infectious Diseases 108
  Resources 124

Chapter 3: Programs and Organizations Related
  to Migrant Farmworkers 139

Chapter 4: Language Resources...147
  Spanish Language..147
  Haitian Creole Language 158

Chapter 5: Policies Affecting Migrant Farmworkers'
  Children 161
  Fair Labor Standards Act 161
  Migrant Health Programs 162
  Medicaid 163
  Vaccines for Children 172
  Special Supplemental Nutrition Program for Women,
    Infants, and Children (WIC)..172

Policies Regarding Foster Care, Adoption,
and Children With Special Needs......................................173
State Children's Health Insurance Program (SCHIP) 174
School Entry 175
Resources 179

Tables and Figure

Tables

Table 1-1. Differences Between United States
and Mexico Educational Systems...35

Table 2-1. Mexican Immunization Schedule 56

Table 2-2. Recommended Immunization Schedule for
Children Not Immunized in the First Year of Life.................58

Table 2-3. Recommended Immunizations for Travelers
to Developing Countries..60

Table 2-4. Fluoride Supplement Prescribing Protocols 74

Table 2-5. Examples of Organophosphate (OP)
and N-methyl Carbamate Pesticides (C) 90

Table 2-6. Signs and Symptoms Associated
With Increasing Methemoglobinemia 94

Table 5-1. Conditions for Medicaid Eligibility 167

Figure

Figure 1-1. Migration Patterns 3

Foreword

For more than 70 years, the American Academy of Pediatrics (AAP) has sought to improve the physical, mental, and social health of all infants, children, adolescents, and young adults. In June 1995, the Academy released the policy statement "Health Care for Children of Farmworker Families," to address the health issues particular to the children of migrant and seasonal farmworkers. Authored by the AAP Committee on Community Health Services (COCHS), this statement discusses how the poverty, lack of health insurance, and mobile lifestyles that most migrant families face can adversely affect the health status of their children. To provide further guidance to pediatricians wishing to implement the recommendations from that statement, the Academy, in partnership with the Migrant Clinicians Network (MCN), has developed *Guidelines for the Care of Migrant Farmworkers' Children.* Used appropriately, the guidelines enable the provision of care that is of high quality and tailored to the context in which children of migrant farmworkers live.

This manual would not have been possible without the expert guidance and constant oversight of Jennie McLaurin, MD, the liaison from the MCN to the COCHS. We are grateful to her and to the staff at MCN. The AAP Board of Directors, COCHS, and many individual members of several AAP committees also played a large role in the success of this project. We also would like to thank and recognize Whole Foods Market for their financial support of the guidelines.

Until we address the unequal access to health care of children of seasonal and migrant farmworkers, it is unlikely that the disparities in health that exist for these children will be erased. However, we are confident that this manual will greatly help those who do care for this unique group of children, and as such will assist in improving their health outcomes. The AAP Committee on Community Health Services is very pleased to have been a part of the publication of this manual.

Paul Melinkovich, MD, Chairperson
AAP Committee on Community Health Services

Purpose and Use of the Manual

The American Academy of Pediatrics (AAP) and the Migrant Clinicians Network (MCN) have jointly produced this manual to assist pediatricians and other primary care professionals in the delivery of comprehensive health care to the children of migrant farmworkers in the United States. It is the goal of the Academy and the MCN that every child of migrant farmworkers have access to a medical home.[1] To reach this goal, a large number of health professionals must be involved. Federally funded migrant health programs have the capacity to serve only 20% of the targeted population; therefore, private practitioners, public health department clinicians, and medical center physicians must be prepared to meet the special needs of migrant farmworkers' children.

This manual describes the unique characteristics of migrant farmworkers' children and assists the clinician with the recognition and treatment of the most common health care needs of this population. The **Understanding the Cultural Context** section in Chapter 1 introduces a cross-cultural medical approach that facilitates understanding of the child's environment. Information on programs, organizations, and publications useful for helping the children of migrant farmworkers is included at the end of each section and in the chapter titled **Programs and Organizations Related to Migrant Farmworkers** (Chapter 3).

The treatment guidelines augment the provision of routine pediatric care, particularly for the reader who does not spend the majority of his or her practice in a migrant health setting. The **Health Care Guidelines** (Chapter 2) are organized for use in ambulatory pediatric settings. Each guideline contains a brief overview of the problems in the setting of the migrant child, important components of the medical history and physical examination, pertinent laboratory data, and considerations in treatment and health education.

Although the policy arena is in continual change, **Policies Affecting Migrant Farmworkers' Children** (Chapter 5) gives an overview that will aid clinicians in their awareness of the basic legislative and legal issues surrounding farm work and migrant workers.

The manual is not meant as a standalone text on the diagnosis and management of common childhood illnesses. All sections deal specifically with conditions as they pertain to children of migrant farmworkers. These guidelines are intended to augment the clinician's knowledge of ambulatory pediatrics in the migrant setting, thereby increasing the capacity to offer children of farmworkers access to community-based, comprehensive, coordinated, and culturally sensitive care.

Reference

1. American Academy of Pediatrics Ad Hoc Task Force on Definition of the Medical Home. The medical home. *Pediatrics*. 1992;90:774

Resources

American Academy of Pediatrics Committee on Community Health Services. Health care for children of farmworker families. *Pediatrics*. 1995;95:952-953

American Academy of Pediatrics Committee on Community Health Services. The pediatrician's role in community pediatrics. *Pediatrics*. 1999;103:1304-1306

Chapter 1: Introduction

Background

As long as there has been large-scale agriculture in the United States, there has been a seasonal labor force employed to cultivate and harvest it. Early reports of migratory farmworkers date to the mid-1800s. Many were immigrant families whose young children worked beside them. At times of national labor shortages, such as during World War II, Congress authorized the solicitation of foreign farm labor, attracting many workers from Mexico. President Truman stated in 1951 that, "We depend on misfortune to build up our force of migratory workers and when the supply is low because there is not enough misfortune at home, we rely on misfortune abroad to replenish the supply."[1]

The Migrant Health Program, Bureau of Primary Health Care, estimates that, nationwide, migrant and seasonal farmworkers and their dependents number between 3 and 5 million (A. Duran, Director, Migrant Health Program Bureau of Primary Health Care, Department of Health and Human Services, oral communication. July 1997). Approximately 1 million of these farmworkers and their dependents are classified as migrant. The term is somewhat arbitrary, as several definitions of "migrant" exist in separate programs and policies.

The Federal Migrant Health Program defines a migrant as one who, in the preceding 24 months, had principal employment in agriculture on a seasonal basis and who moved to seek such employment. The National Agricultural Workers Survey (NAWS) of the US Department of Labor, which is a source of most of the demographic data on farmworkers, defines a migrant as one who travels at least 75 miles to obtain a job in US agriculture. Exact numbers of children of migrant farmworkers are not known, however, more than 600,000 school-age children are enrolled in migrant education programs in 47 of the 50 states.

Children of farmworkers move with their families in three patterns of mobility (Figure 1-1). Most are point-to-point migrants, moving from a home base (83% claim Mexico as home base) to one or more US farm jobs, and then back home again. Employment on the US farm constitutes the majority of the family's annual earnings, and the home base is a strategy to contain costs by residing in inexpensive settings during the off-season. One third of families are nomadic migrants, traveling from crop to crop usually working for at least three employers in two locations in separate states. A small number of nomadic farmworkers travel out of the United States as part of their regular mobility pattern. The third group follows a restricted circuit within a small geographic area, such as the Central Valley in California. Children of farmworkers are thus a part of several communities in terms of schooling, housing, social relationships, and health care professionals. The classic construct of a medical home must be adapted to address the needs of the child within his or her particular pattern of mobility.

The migrant farmworker labor force traditionally has been largely Hispanic. In recent years, the growth of the Hispanic sector in the migrant population has accelerated, such that 94% of migrant farmworkers are, or have family members who are, Hispanic.[3] Most adults (85%) are foreign-born and come from landless poor families in Mexico and Latin America.[2] The average adult foreign-born farmworker has only 7 years of formal education. Women have even fewer years of schooling and often have particular difficulty with written information, whether in Spanish or English. Thus, language is a barrier to providing care in terms of spoken communication and as a resource for education. Forecasting of future farm labor needs indicates that harvest work will continue to be supplied by recent immigrants.

Figure 1-1. Migration Patterns

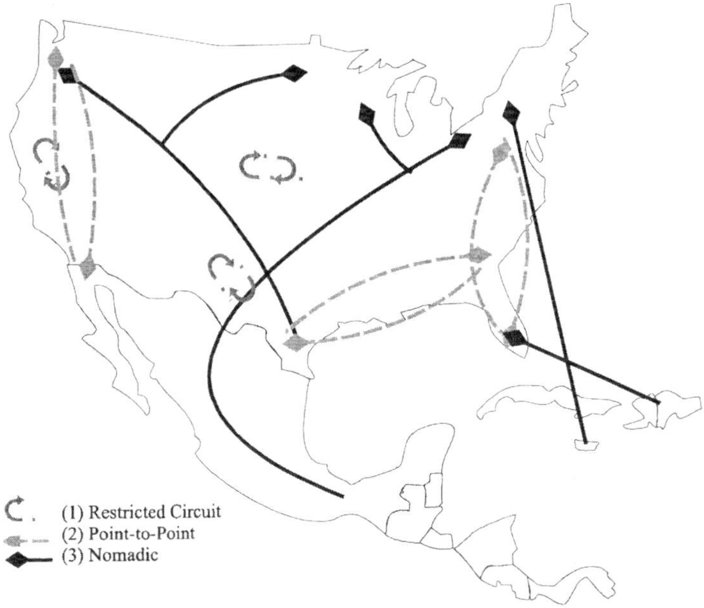

C.   (1) Restricted Circuit
    (2) Point-to-Point
    (3) Nomadic

Reprinted with permission from the Migrant Clinicians Network.

Children of farmworkers often are born in the United States and, therefore, have different citizenship and eligibility for US health and human services than do their parents. While most male farmworkers are documented workers (that is, are legally employed), many of the women do not have authorization for US residence. It has been shown that children who are US citizens in families such as these experience limited access to care based on the restrictions of the undocumented family member. Children of undocumented workers also are much more likely to spend part of each year in their family's native country than are children of documented residents. The community of the migrant child may be a complex blend of two separate worlds.

Farmworker families live in conditions characterized by poverty, unstable housing, unreliable transportation, and social and cultural isolation. Many lack telephones, have no ability to communicate with the local community, and spend at least one third of the year unemployed. The median annual income of a worker is $5,000, whether paid by the piece or by the hour. Despite the presence of multiple wage earners in a family, 73% of migrant children live in poverty. Fewer than 20% use needs-based services, and only 25% of families have any form of third-party payment for health care.[2] In addition to their parents and siblings, children often live with extended family and nonfamily members. The family usually depends on one or more working adult male member for transportation, as most women do not drive, and, typically, public transportation is not available in rural areas. Housing may be located on farm property, exposing the child to agricultural chemicals and workplace hazards. Fewer than 20% of children of migrant farmworkers are enrolled in licensed child care programs, and an unknown number of these children accompany their parents to the field.

There are a number of federally funded programs for migrant farmworkers and their families, including health and educational services. The Migrant Health Program, established in 1962, funds more than 120 community/migrant health centers with 400 sites in 43 states and Puerto Rico. The goal is to provide comprehensive, community-oriented, culturally appropriate primary care services to farmworkers and their dependents. While the services are effective for improving the health of clients served, fewer than 20% of the nation's farmworker families have access to these centers.[1] Therefore, the broader pediatric practice community must provide a medical home to the majority of these children.

No national data exist on child health indicators in the
farmworker population such as rates of infant mortality, birth
defects, adolescent pregnancy, or homicides. However, a profile
of the health status of farmworkers' children can be constructed.
Migrant children receive inadequate preventive medical care,
are exposed to occupational illnesses and injury, have an increased rate of infectious diseases and toxic exposures, an
increased risk of family violence and mental health problems,
and are subject to nutritional and educational deprivation. In
Monitoring Children's Health: Key Indicators, the authors state
that "the major determinants of favorable maternal and child
health status relate to quality-of-life issues: nurture, social
supports, nutrition, housing, and education."[3] The potential
for each of these determinants to be experienced in full is
thwarted by the environment of migrant life.

Understanding the Cultural Context

Overview of Cross-Cultural Medicine

It is important to recognize how differences in language, health beliefs, expectations of care, communication styles, and access to resources impact our clinical encounters. Migrant farmworkers are often from different ethnic and racial groups than their health care professionals, but although these may constitute the most visible contrasts, they are not necessarily the most important. One of the biggest contrasts between the health care provider and migrant farmworker families lies in the disparity in socioeconomic status. This factor alone may be the most crucial in shaping the clinical interaction. Most health care professionals have experiences in "cross-cultural medicine" because they treat patients of different genders, religions, ages, and backgrounds. The same principles of openness, compassion, and active listening that characterize any successful clinical encounter will serve clinicians well as the range of differences between them and their patients widens.

Cross-cultural medicine can be complex for the health care team, but consider the farmworkers' perspective — they are involved in a doubly complex cross-cultural experience as they deal with the subculture of biomedicine. The health care system with its distinct language ("medical jargon") and cultural rules (medical students are the ones wearing short white coats) is confusing for many patients. Additionally, biomedicine's unique health belief model may be foreign and unacceptable to individuals outside of our subculture. For example, biomedicine is infused with the notion of a mind-body dichotomy — either you have a "real" disease or it is "all in your head." This distinction is not made in other health belief models. Awareness that individual health beliefs are indeed culturally determined and not scientific fact may help the clinician be more open to the cultural beliefs of others.

Language

_What the scalpel is to the surgeon, words are to the
clinician... the conversation between doctor and patient
is the heart of the practice of medicine._ P. Tumulty

Overcoming language barriers is the single most important
challenge in cross-cultural medicine. When patients or their families speak a foreign language, the most critical first step is to ensure that an appropriate interpreter is used. Guidelines for select-
ing and working with interpreters are covered in this manual in
the section titled Bilingual Interpreters in the Clinical Setting.
The ability to establish rapport with patients does not have to be
negatively affected by the presence of an interpreter, and communication can be enhanced if interpreters are used appropriately as
partners in the interaction. Even among people speaking the same
language, communication problems can arise. Be sensitive to the
fact that a patient's use of words and their associated meanings
may be different from your own. African-American farmworkers
may refer to problems with "blood," meaning anemia ("low
blood"), high blood pressure ("high blood"), or syphilis ("bad
blood"). Asking for clarification or more information is always
a good idea.

The need to avoid medical jargon may seem self-evident,
but it is sometimes difficult to appreciate the extent to which
our speech is filled with technical terminology foreign to our
patients. An example of this occurred when a patient who was
informed that her HIV test was "positive" initially reacted as if
this was a "positive" or good thing. It is easy to use confusing,
technical language without realizing it.

What is not said may prove to be as important as what is said
during some clinical encounters. In Hispanic cultures there are
taboos about discussing certain subjects, such as sexuality, especially with members of the opposite sex. Trained interpreters can
help to address delicate subjects in a culturally sensitive manner.

If discussion of a sensitive issue is needed for the evaluation of a patient, acknowledge his or her discomfort with the topic, and then explain why the information is needed before proceeding.

Cultural conventions in expressing respect toward physicians may prevent patients or their families from verbalizing concerns or questions about treatment provided. Patients may not directly challenge a physician even if they disagree with the diagnosis or treatment plan. Do not misread a passive, smiling face as a sign of agreement. Give permission for open discussion by specifically asking if there are any areas of disagreement. This is especially true among vulnerable populations. Patients or their families may be embarrassed to admit that they do not understand instructions or that they do not have the resources to comply with them. Do not assume that a family understands just because they do not ask questions. Be proactive in soliciting questions from patients and in determining areas of misunderstanding.

Suggestions for Improving the Communication of Treatment Plans

1. Have the patient or parent repeat the instructions back to you.

2. Provide simple, concrete instructions. "Bring him back right away if he develops a fever higher than 102°F" is more clear than "Come back if he isn't better."

3. Demonstrations are more effective than explanations. Show parents how to measure correct doses of medicine or how to take a rectal temperature.

4. Written instructions or patient education materials can reinforce verbal messages. Make sure these are written at very low literacy levels (3rd to 4th grade).

5. Do not rely solely on written materials for explaining key points. Many migrant farmworkers are functionally illiterate and may not feel comfortable admitting an inability to read.

Perceptions of Time and Measurement

Because many migrant farmworkers do not have extensive formal education, the use of numeric scales and concepts may be confusing. Asking patients to describe pain on a scale from 1 to 10, for example, may be inappropriate. The representations in visual aids like graphs should be carefully explained. For example, some clinicians refer to the growth chart as "the road to health," therefore, parents understand that their child needs to stay on "the road." Graphs depicting appropriate times for childhood vaccines or growth charts also can be confusing for individuals without formal math skills. Demonstrate the use of a digital thermometer if accurate recording of temperatures is necessary.

Differences in the way the patient and the health care provider perceive the concept of time can cause frustration between both parties. One area that may cause conflict is the notion of chronic illnesses. Many migrant farmworkers, regardless of ethnicity, have a health belief model that focuses on perceived symptoms as defining illness states. They may have difficulty believing they have a disease (diabetes, hypertension, or asthma) when they feel well. Additionally, the idea that they have a disease that cannot be cured but must be managed over time may feel very foreign to them. Physicians may become irritated with patients who only take medication for a short period, fail to return for follow-up visits, "doctor shop," and/or try alternative healers in efforts to cure their disease. Understanding that these actions arise from difficulty in understanding or accepting the idea of disease chronicity should prompt physicians to explain and reinforce this concept repeatedly over time.

Social Organization

The culture of the United States places great emphasis on individuals. The US Constitution discusses the rights of individual citizens, and the importance of patient autonomy is central to Western medical ethics. Migrant farmworkers from more traditional cultures place less emphasis on individualism and more on group harmony and collective decision making. Mothers may feel uncomfortable making even seemingly minor decisions about their children's health without first discussing things with their husbands or extended family members. Thus, it is important to establish a professional relationship with the entire family. If a grandmother continually gives advice that undermines your treatment plans, do not simply tell the parents to ignore her. Invite her to the next clinic visit and negotiate a treatment plan that everyone in the family supports. Hierarchy and respect are important within many family structures. Disrupting this hierarchy may make patients feel uncomfortable. Having a teenager translate for his parents, for example, may embarrass them because it reverses the usual lines of authority.

The crew leader (or the farmworker's supervisor), although not a family member, should be involved to some degree in treatment plans because he often controls a family's access to housing, transportation, and time off work. As an employer, the crew leader should never be allowed to dictate therapeutic decisions and should not have access to confidential patient information. It is almost always inappropriate for crew leaders to be present during patient encounters as interpreters or observers. However, once a treatment plan has been defined by the clinician and the family, relevant aspects of the treatment plan should be communicated by the physician to the crew leader. Crew leaders are much more receptive to instructions from a physician than from a farmworker. If the crew leader has accompanied the family to the visit, the physician should personally address the issue of resources with the crew leader: "Juan's mother will need a week off from work to care for him, and you will need to transport them back to the clinic on Tuesday for a dressing change." A written list of instructions for the crew leader, signed by the physician, may be sent home with the family if the crew leader is unavailable.

Parenting Beliefs

Parenting practices vary greatly among cultures, and it is important for health professionals to carefully examine the objective evidence that favors one practice over another. Often our advice and recommendations to parents are based more on our own cultural understanding of appropriate parenting than on scientific evidence. Recognizing this, the health professional should tolerate and respect other cultural beliefs unless they are known to be detrimental to the child's health, development, or sense of self-worth.

Breastfeeding

Many migrant women choose to breastfeed their babies, and they do so for the same reasons other women breastfeed: they believe it is better for their babies. Our culture sends mixed messages to women about breastfeeding that may influence or encourage farmworkers to use infant formula. Advertising and media images promoting formula feeding, and the availability of free formula through the Special Supplemental Nutrition Program for Women, Infants, and Children (WIC) and from hospital gift packs make bottle feeding seem like a more acceptable alternative. To counterbalance this misinformation, education regarding the benefits of breastfeeding should be provided early in prenatal care and reinforced by health professionals over time. Given the paternalistic social structure of many Hispanic families, involving fathers in individual discussions about infant feeding is important. Feelings of embarrassment are especially important issues for Hispanic women, so specific instruction about how to nurse discreetly should be given. One migrant health center successfully increased their rates of breastfeeding initiation by arranging prenatal breastfeeding classes using free infant layettes as incentives for attendance. Breastfeeding was presented as particularly convenient for the migrant lifestyle because of the ease of traveling with a breastfed infant in contrast to the "difficulty of providing clean, refrigerated formula on long car trips." The advantage of fewer episodes of illness necessitating long waiting times at a clinic also was stressed.

Persuading a migrant family to initiate breastfeeding is not nearly as difficult as providing support for maintaining breastfeeding for a minimum of 1 year as recommended by the American Academy of Pediatrics.[4] Breastfeeding may be difficult for migrant women for several reasons. They often are separated from close friends and family members to whom they would traditionally turn for lactation advice. Ensure that women are comfortable breastfeeding and know correct breastfeeding techniques before they leave the hospital by providing access to bilingual lactation consultants or nurses or by providing translation support for monolingual clinicians. Nurses and other health staff may find it difficult to provide teaching and support with every feeding to non–English-speaking mothers because of the inconvenience involved in summoning a translator or their own discomfort with the language barrier. Problem solving with the nurses and other staff is the key to identifying solutions to these barriers to care.

Logistical concerns after hospital discharge also may limit the duration of breastfeeding. Some women return to work in the fields very soon after delivery out of economic necessity. Finding the time or a private place to express milk is difficult when a woman is part of a busy field crew. One solution may be to teach the woman to discreetly express her milk manually every few hours while working. The physician or other staff member should spend time with nursing mothers to problem solve how to overcome the unique barriers farmworker women may have in maintaining breastfeeding.

**Strategies for Encouraging Breastfeeding
in Migrant Families**

1. Hire a bilingual medical assistant or other staff member who is cross-trained to provide basic lactation advice and maternal postnatal instructions.

2. Hire a translator dedicated to the obstetrics floor.

3. Use bilingual visiting nurses or community health nurses to reinforce breastfeeding messages after discharge.

4. Purchase Spanish-language videotapes (La Leche League International is one good source) to supplement one-on-one teaching.

5. Provide, prenatally, non–English-speaking women with identification cards that indicate their intent to breastfeed. These cards can be presented to labor and delivery staff on admission.

6. Design pictorial flip charts that patients can use to indicate their request that their baby be brought in for breastfeeding.

7. Train volunteer lay health advisors (mothers who have experience with breastfeeding and parenting) who can "adopt" a new mother and provide advice over time.

Infant Feeding

Infant feeding practices may vary between ethnic groups. Many Hispanic mothers introduce solids at a very young age, even 2 weeks of age, in the belief that their children are not satisfied with milk only. Given the poor sanitary conditions of many migrant camps, feeding anything but breast milk during the first few months of life places babies at risk for diarrheal or gastrointestinal illnesses. Reviewing with parents the nutritional information on baby food jars (indicating that they are mostly water and actually have fewer calories and fat than milk) may help to convince them that milk is more nutritious. For parents who insist on introducing solids, encourage them to use dried, fortified rice cereal mixed with boiled water or breast milk. Most parents are attracted to this feeding plan once they are informed that cereals have more iron and vitamins, which they recognize as important in preventing anemia.

Food may be used by some migrant families to reward or placate children. Infants or children may be offered food every time they cry, and infant crying may be interpreted as indicating hunger. Sweets are used liberally, especially by extended family members or family friends, as small tokens of affection or to bribe children. These displays of indulgence may be harmful to children's teeth or may lead to obesity. Practitioners worried about early childhood caries (ECC) from nighttime bottles can suggest alternate methods of calming a crying baby. For older children, alternative treats (stickers, crayons) can take the place of candy.

A healthy baby is often envisioned as a chubby baby by Hispanics. Many families tend to overfeed infants and children in the belief that this will make them more resistant to disease. During the toddler period, as children's appetites tend to decrease, many parents become distressed. "No appetite" is a common complaint. A good approach is to reassure parents that this is a normal trait for children of this age and to show them how the child is continuing to grow well. Because some families will begin to offer sweets or juices in a desperate effort to entice their toddler to eat *anything,* it is wise to encourage them to continue to offer nutritious foods frequently during the day. Vitamins are believed to enhance the appetite of children, and many parents will ask for advice about their use during this age. Recommendations on the use of vitamins should take into account the expense for a family on a limited budget. There is really no other reason to discourage the use of vitamins as a placebo appetite enhancer as long as they are secured in a childproof container.

The cultural value placed on obesity among children may make it difficult to address. In a culture that supports the idea of overweight children as healthy and loved, it seems incongruous for a physician to indicate that a child is too heavy. One way to address this issue in a culturally acceptable way is to draw on the Hispanic notion of balance. Excesses in many areas of life are viewed as unhealthy. If you begin by acknowledging the cultural belief that thin children are not healthy, but point out that excessively obese children also are unhealthy, you may be able to convince the family of the need to obtain balance in the area of weight. Diabetes, common among Hispanics, can be used effectively as an example of an obesity-related disease outcome.

Child Discipline

Discipline practices vary widely across and within cultures. Any generalizations about the way farmworkers discipline their children must be viewed with caution. The most useful information for the clinician will come from personal conversations with the family. You may observe that families are more tolerant of exuberant play activities in clinic waiting rooms. Bribery or displaced threats may be used to control behavior. It is fairly common to hear comments such as "be quiet or the doctor is going to give you a shot," during clinic visits. This type of interaction should be discouraged because they often result in frightened, uncooperative patients. Paradoxically, corporal punishment may be used even through the teenage years.

Many parents are aware of child abuse statutes in this country but are confused about how to discipline their children in this culture without breaking the law. The pediatrician can play an important role in supporting parents' need to discipline their children while teaching them effective ways to do so. Begin by negotiating mutually acceptable, consistent discipline strategies with families, realizing that they may not be comfortable with high-control styles. The concept of "time out" is foreign to most migrant parents, but may be accepted if the idea is reinforced over several visits as trust is established. If parents do not accept the idea of "time out," plan other discipline strategies with the parents. Advice on how to effectively discipline adolescents without the use of corporal punishment is often well received. Some communities have organized classes for parents who may have particular problems dealing with their children as they become acculturated.

In regard to expectations of childhood development, some Hispanic families place more emphasis on a preschooler's social skills, such as obedience and establishing rapport with peers, than other developmental achievements. Although this is adaptive in their cultural context, it may place farmworker children at a disadvantage educationally in this country. Strategies for improving school readiness should be specifically addressed with anticipatory guidance. *(See School Readiness in Chapter 2.)*

Health Belief Model

Hispanic farmworkers often share a health belief model that differs from biomedicine. The etiology of disease often is not understood in terms of the germ theory or other biomedical constructs. Illness may be believed to have spiritual causes such as curses, demonic possession, or exposure to moonlight or nocturnal airs. Severe stress, overwork, a psychological shock, or family disharmony may lead to illness. Expectations of care are based on health belief models, and patients are likely to be noncompliant with treatment plans if they seem incongruous with their belief system.

Farmworkers may believe in theories of "hot" and "cold" in disease causation. For example, some may believe that drinking ice water or eating "cold" foods such as melons (the classification of foods does not necessarily refer to temperature) after working in the hot fields may cause disease. This belief may complicate the treatment of fever as parents may be loathe to undress or bathe febrile children for fear they will worsen an illness. Explaining cooling measures in mechanical terms ("they help to draw out the infection") is often more acceptable to parents than trying to substitute beliefs about the cause and meaning of fever.

Ideas about appropriate treatment may include a preference for injectable drugs over oral forms of medicine. Injections are regarded as stronger, faster acting, and definitive therapy as opposed to oral medications, which are viewed as weaker or palliative.

Culture-bound syndromes are illness complexes that exist only within a particular culture. Premenstrual syndrome (PMS) is an example of a culture-bound syndrome accepted by most health care professionals in our society. It is an illness, however, that has been recognized only in certain developed, Western countries since World War II. Culture-bound syndromes described by farmworkers are experienced as "real" illnesses, just as PMS is understood and experienced as real by participants in our culture. It is inappropriate to suggest to a family that such illnesses do not exist. When necessary, negotiate a reinterpretation of the illness experience into a form that the practitioner and family agree will lead to optimal treatment of the child. For example, "Your child does not have *caída de la mollera* (sunken fontanel) at this time, just mild dehydration and diarrhea. We can use oral rehydration solution to prevent her from developing caída. At home, I want you to watch the appearance of her fontanel. You also need to look for other signs of dehydration. If she does develop *caída de la mollera,* we will admit her to the hospital. How does that sound to you?"

Culture-bound Syndromes That May Be Encountered in Pediatric Practice*

Caída de la mollera (sunken fontanel). A disease exclusively of young infants. Symptoms also may include diarrhea or lethargy. This is considered a serious, even life-threatening, condition. Treatment consists of massage of the hard palate and holding the child upside down.

Susto. May affect people of all ages. It is caused by a severe fright (eg, unexpectedly encountering an aggressive, barking dog). Vague symptoms of decreased appetite, personality change, and inability to concentrate may last for up to a year. Folk healers are generally sought for treatment.

Mal de ojo (evil eye). May be caused inadvertently (by a drunken man, for example) or purposely (by a vengeful neighbor). The curse applied continues to cause health problems until it is removed by a layperson or folk healer. Symptoms vary, but could include pain syndromes, failure to thrive, and lethargy.

Empacho. A condition in which food becomes stuck in the intestines causing a blockage. It is caused by overeating, eating the wrong kinds of foods, or mixing infant formula with milk. Symptoms include nausea, diarrhea, stomach cramps, and a lump in the abdomen. It is treated with herbal teas, abdominal massage, and a restricted diet at home or in combination with a folk healer's care.

* Folk illnesses vary slightly among different Hispanic subgroups and among different regions, so variations among patients are to be expected.

Explanatory Model Approach

Explanatory models are a set of beliefs used by all patients to explain their illness. Although it is possible to paint with broad strokes a picture of migrants' health beliefs and practices, clinicians need to move beyond stereotypes and generalizations when interacting with individual patients. A patient-centered approach to health care that elicits explanatory models is probably the most helpful skill in cross-cultural practice. The health beliefs of migrant workers are shaped by their culture, but it is important to recognize that we are all individuals. Culture is only one factor that influences our illness experiences. The following case example illustrates the utility of this approach:

> Maria-Elena was a 15-year-old Hispanic farmworker who presented with a history of headaches for the past 4 years. The headaches occurred on the left side, were throbbing, and were sometimes associated with nausea. They were not associated with neurologic symptoms or a preceding aura. They occurred on an almost daily basis and were relieved when she went into her dark bedroom to sleep for a few hours. Her physical examination was completely normal. A biomedical assessment at this stage pointed to the diagnosis of migraine headache. Treatment would have included medicines for headache prophylaxis and acute episodes of pain. Using an explanatory model approach, the patient was, however, questioned further.
>
> Maria-Elena indicated that her headaches were so severe that she had not attended school in more than 6 months. She believed her headaches were caused by beatings she had received on her head from her grandmother. She believed the headaches had worsened over the past year as punishment for her ambivalence over her grandmother's recent death. The stress of her recent immigration from Guatemala and her social isolation also seemed to contribute to her illness. Her main

fear was that she had suffered permanent damage to her head, and would eventually die from her condition. She was initially worried that discussing these problems would worsen her symptoms, as they triggered long crying spells. She did not want pain medication because she did not believe it would help cure her problem. In fact, she already had been seen by several other doctors over the past few months. She felt they did not understand the nature of her problem, so she was noncompliant with their treatment regimens. What she wanted was a way to escape her perpetual punishment as well as someone to listen to her story and help work through her complex emotions.

At this stage, the connection between her past abuse as the cause of the headaches was explicitly acknowledged. She and her family were referred to a bilingual counselor for further therapy. The sacraments of the conciliation ("confession") and anointing of the sick were agreed on as the means to receive forgiveness for her anger and hatred toward her dead grandmother and to begin definitive spiritual and physical healing. These sacraments were arranged through a local Catholic church, where Maria-Elena became involved in a Hispanic youth group. In addition, information was given about migraine headaches. Eventually, we were able to negotiate an explanatory model that defined chronic migraine headaches as the residual physical sequelae of her beatings. At that time, Maria-Elena was receptive to medical treatment of her now less frequent and less disabling migraines.

Using an explanatory model approach resulted in a more effective treatment plan and improved patient satisfaction and compliance.

Helpful Questions to Elicit Patients' Explanatory Models

- What is the name of your problem?
- What caused it?
- Why did it start when it did?
- What will this problem do to your body?
- How has this illness affected your life?
- What worries you most about this problem?
- What are your expectations? What kind of treatment do you think you need?
- Are there other things you want (support, reassurance, or explanations)?

Self-care

Self-care is used for 70% to 90% of all illness episodes in every culture. Understanding the differences in self-care techniques among cultures is important for the clinician to appreciate. Below are some issues that may arise in relation to self-care treatments common in Hispanic populations.

- Treatments used for self-care may involve biologically active substances such as antibiotics and vitamins.

- In Mexico, it is possible to buy a variety of oral and injectable medicines without a prescription. Up to 20% of Hispanic migrant farmworkers have self-injected medicines, often using shared needles.[5] This practice continues in the United States, and it is important to ask specifically whether these treatments are being used in children.

- Medicinal preparations used among Hispanic groups in the United States have been found to contain high levels of lead or mercury.

- Common home remedies used in Hispanic culture include various herbal teas. Some herbs can be toxic, so it is advisable to ask specifically about these treatments.

- Cupping is a form of self-treatment that may leave marks that can be confused with child abuse. A heated glass is placed on the child's skin. As it cools, a slight suction is generated against the skin that "draws out the infection." Repeated cupping may cause slight bruising over the round area circumscribed by the glass.

- Other forms of self-treatment in Hispanic cultures consist of rituals involving eggs or religious symbols such as crosses or candles.

There may be some reluctance or embarrassment on the part of the family to discuss these types of therapy. A nonjudgmental approach to such disclosures is warranted to facilitate trust and openness in other areas of communication.

Folk Health Care
Patients may use informal, complementary healers either prior to or concurrently with their encounters with physicians. Some of these healers are available to migrant farmworkers living in the United States. It is important to respect the legitimacy of these complementary healers, and to try to work with them when possible. On the other hand, information about the specific treatments suggested by these healers should be elicited to ensure that they do not represent a physical or psychological hazard to a child. Also, parents should be cautioned not to abandon necessary medical treatments on the advice of these other healers.

Informal Healers in the Hispanic Culture

Curanderos or the Puerto Rican equivalent, *santinguadoras* or *espiritistas,* are healers most often sought for help with folk illnesses such as those mentioned previously. They use a variety of treatments, including massage and quasi-religious rituals, to effect a cure.

Sobadores or bone setters act somewhat like physical thera-pists or orthopaedists to treat mechanical musculoskeletal injuries. The term is sometimes used interchangeably with curandero.

Brujos or witches are healers who use a variety of magical powers to influence the spiritual world that affects health.

Professional Health Care in Mexico

Many physicians have questions about the health care systems in their patients' countries of origin. Like the United States, Mexico does not have universal health insurance, and access and quality of care vary depending on economic status and loca-tion. Employees of the government, including teachers, receive medical benefits often at special, designated hospitals and clin-ics. Private physicians see patients at rates that are less expensive than in the United States but that are too costly for many fami-lies to afford. Public clinics are available, but care received there is often perceived as substandard and may involve very long waits. In rural areas, inexperienced physicians-in-training may provide care during required service rotations.

Treating patients in a binational setting presents certain chal-lenges. In general, it is impossible to obtain copies of medical records from Mexico through the mail. If medical records are indispensable, the best alternative may be to have a relative or friend in the home country obtain the information in person, and then forward it to an address in the United States. Identification of prescription drugs obtained in Mexico can be difficult because they include medicines and brand names not available in this country. Some patients who take medicines for chronic conditions prefer to obtain their medicines in Mexico, where they can be purchased for a lower price. Identifying those drugs can be a challenge. A book equivalent to the *Physicians' Desk Reference,* called *Diccionario de Especialidades Farmacéuticas,* is available for purchase from the National Center for Farmworker Health Resource Center. Some poison control centers also can be a resource for drug identification. Another service, Call Our Pharmacist, helps to identify foreign drugs for a fee. *(See Resources.)*

Practicing Within the Social Context

Another challenge of cross-cultural medicine is understanding and negotiating the complex social context in which healing takes place. Farmworkers share many of the same problems as other families of low socioeconomic status in this country. However, there are some stressors that are unique to this population. Farmworkers are often extremely isolated from their extended families and friends and from the non-migrant residents in their communities. Local institutions, such as churches, schools, and recreation centers, often view migrants as outsiders. Racism in many communities can add to the atmosphere of distance or hostility. Ambivalence about cultural identity often is an issue for migrant farmworkers who live in two different cultures. When children assimilate to a new culture faster than their parents, conflict can develop within the family. These stressors contribute to the context in which illness develops and health care is received.

Providing a Medical Home: Barriers and Strategies

Financial barriers to care are significant for farmworker families. Virtually none have private insurance coverage, and despite their low-income levels, many are not eligible for Medicaid coverage due to welfare reform legislation. Even those who do have coverage have difficulty with the portability of Medicaid coverage during migration from state to state. Also, because they are not permanent residents of one state or county, migrant farmworkers have difficulty meeting the eligibility criteria for public and private assistance programs. Migrant health centers serve the needs of thousands of farmworkers each year, but they are not available in all communities. Community physicians, health departments, clinics, and community health centers may be called on during the migrant season to help farmworker children without other access to care.

Other access problems for migrant farmworkers include limited transportation and time off from work. Ways to accommodate their special circumstances include flexibility in scheduling, such as allowing patients to set appointment times to match unreliable transportation (eg, "sometime Monday morning"). Evening or weekend appointments may be especially convenient. To decrease the need for multiple return visits, health care providers can offer preventive services such as immunizations when patients present in the clinic for acute care.

Be aware that contacting migrant families at home may be difficult, as few have telephones or mailing addresses. Empirical therapy often makes more sense in this setting than withholding treatment pending the results of lab tests. For example, it is rarely helpful to obtain throat cultures because, by the time cultures are positive, the patient is unavailable for treatment. When this is not medically feasible, try to arrange for family members to contact your clinic at a specified time. If possible, obtain the telephone number of a crew leader or the farmer as a backup.

For a variety of reasons, migrant farmworkers may have difficulty negotiating complex systems in this country. It is important to recognize how easy it is for a migrant child to get "lost" or "fall through the cracks" when referred to a large medical center. Establish a contact person who can serve as a patient advocate or caseworker either within your office or at another agency.

Strategies for Improving Comprehensive Care

1. Develop payment plans or sliding scale fees based on income.

2. Ask residents, retired physicians, and pediatric consultants to donate small amounts of time.

3. Use drug samples, generic medicines, and inexpensive home remedies whenever appropriate.

4. Solicit medications from pharmaceutical companies, most of which will donate 3- to 6-month supplies of medication for chronic conditions in children demonstrating financial need.

5. Always provide the family with a portable medical record detailing, at a minimum, immunization, growth, allergy, and laboratory data.

6. Consider designing a Community Access to Child Health (CATCH) program. *(See Resources.)*

7. Contact employers of farmworkers to solicit help in promoting access to care.

Migration and Discontinuity

Continuity with a health care professional is recognized as essential in the delivery of quality care. Many migrant families are able to establish surprisingly stable relationships with physicians over time as they return at regular intervals to the same communities. Still, interruption in the continuity of care is common and must be anticipated.

Strategies for Adapting Health Care to the Lifestyle of Migrant Children

1. Provide vaccinations and preventive services at the time of acute visits.

2. Provide patients with copies of the medical record including their vaccination record and growth chart.

3. Stress to parents the importance of bringing all medications and immunization records to every clinic (or emergency department) visit.

4. Ask parents about their planned length of stay in your area and their future travel itinerary.

5. Provide the name, address, and telephone number of clinics, physicians, and schools at their next destination.

Bilingual Interpreters in the Clinical Setting

More than 31 million persons currently living in the United States do not speak English.[9,10] A greater number of individuals have limited English proficiency that seriously restricts their ability to communicate with health care professionals. Physicians increasingly provide services to patients and families who speak little or no English. Correctly diagnosing, treating, and providing education to these patients requires the assistance of an interpreter. Interpreters are equally important in situations where the patient or family speaks some English but still may not understand health terms and may have difficulty in accurately describing symptoms and providing the health history. Clinicians need only contemplate the difficulties they encounter daily in obtaining accurate medical histories from patients whose first language is English to appreciate the potential problems of communicating with someone whose command of the English language is limited. Health care professionals are dealing with a bicultural as well as a bilingual situation. They will need assistance in understanding the nuances of language and culture that can make a critical difference in communicating with patients and providing appropriate health care.

A large percentage of the migrant farmworker population in this country immigrated to the United States from Mexico and Central America, and many speak little or no English. Though the majority speak Spanish, there are a small number of farmworker families who speak Indian languages, as well as farmworkers from Haiti who speak Creole. Providing printed materials and instructions in Spanish or Creole cannot replace the need for interpreter services. Many farmworkers lack sufficient literacy skills to understand printed materials in their own language, and relying on printed materials does not provide any opportunity for the patient or parent to ask questions and clarify information.

Please note: Certified interpreters for the deaf are necessary when providing care for hearing-impaired patients familiar with sign language. The information in this section is limited to concerns relating to bilingual interpreters only.

The Ideal Situation: A Trained Interpreter

Physicians generally recognize the importance of using an interpreter when communication problems exist. However, many physicians fail to appreciate the importance of using a trained or professional interpreter rather than relying on family and friends of the patient to interpret critical health information. Health care professionals may falsely assume that interpreting is a fairly simple task for anyone understanding two languages. However, interpreting is a highly complex process requiring the bilingual individual to make critical choices related to conveying complicated information between individuals of different languages and cultures.[6] Effective interpretation requires a high degree of fluency in both languages, a knowledge of the regional idiomatic differences that exist within a single language, and familiarity with both cultures. In the case of clinical interpretation, knowledge of medical terms and confidentiality are critical.

Trained interpreters should be used whenever any degree of language barrier exists. The use of unskilled interpreters leads to inadequate translation of medical complaints, diagnoses, and instructions.[7,8] A potential liability issue exists for physicians failing to use a trained interpreter when needed by their patients.

What Is a Trained Interpreter?

The trained bilingual interpreter demonstrates a high level of fluency in both languages and is skilled in the various techniques of interpretation. The trained interpreter is aware of the many idiomatic differences among Spanish-speaking persons from different areas and countries and is aware of cultural differences that may affect the communication process. The trained interpreter understands the serious nature of the interpreter's role in the communication process and does not filter information. Trained interpreters recognize their skill limitations and inform the health care professional when the information to be translated is beyond their capabilities. Interpreters trained to work in a medical setting understand the importance of confidentiality of patient information.

Clinicians who are not bilingual have difficulty in determining the interpreting skill of an applicant and have no way of determining whether an interpreter is performing adequately. For this reason, standards are helpful in ensuring that the interpreter meets the minimum criteria for interpreter skills. Trained or professional interpreters may have a variety of credentials and training. With the exception of federal court interpreters, there are no national standards or credentials for medical interpreters.

Other factors also may be important in choosing an interpreter. Using an interpreter from the same country of the patient is often helpful. There are many stories of misunderstandings that occur between Spanish-speaking individuals from different countries. Ordinary words may have different and sometimes obscene and offensive meanings in different Spanish-speaking countries.[7] Class and cultural differences also may make patients uncomfortable and communication more difficult. Many patients are not comfortable if the interpreter is not the same gender. With younger children this may not be an issue, but it becomes more important with teenage patients and adults.

Desirable Qualifications for Interpreters

- A college degree in the foreign language or equivalent education and experience
- Advanced oral and written skills in both languages
- Cross-cultural training and experience
- Knowledge of medical terms, training in ethical issues, and experience in interpretation

---

Why Not Use a Family Member or Friend to Interpret?

Physicians who use bilingual family members or friends to interpret are taking a serious risk, as they have no assurance as to the interpreter's competency in either language. Also, family members may filter information or may answer without asking the patient. There are additional concerns that patients may be uncomfortable in responding to sensitive questions in the presence of a family member or friend. The patient, dependent on family or friends to interpret, has no assurance of the confidentiality of the health information they provide or receive from the physician.

The practice of using a bilingual child as an interpreter for the family is highly discouraged because it places an inappropriate burden of responsibility on the child and demonstrates a lack of respect for the parents. This is particularly true when sensitive information is discussed. Using a child as interpreter has been shown to seriously affect the quality and quantity of information conveyed to and from the adult.[8]

In some situations, health care professionals rely on a staff member with limited foreign language skills to interpret. Again, this is a risky alternative since there is no assurance as to the accuracy of the transfer of important health information. Using unqualified interpreters has resulted in serious miscommunications with farmworker patients. For example, in one such situation a family thought they were supposed to administer lice medication orally to their children rather than apply it topically.

I Know Some Spanish, Why Do I Need to Use an Interpreter?

Some clinicians may rely on academic training in Spanish or may take a quick medical interpretation course. Evaluations suggest that significant errors occur when these health care professionals attempt to care for Spanish-speaking patients without the assistance of a trained interpreter. Medical language courses may be a useful adjunct to interpreters, but they do not replace them.[11] Effective communication requires a high level of fluency in both languages.

How Do I Find a Trained Interpreter?

Difficulty in finding a trained interpreter will vary from community to community. Areas with large numbers of immigrant populations are generally better resources for bilingual individuals with the necessary interpreting skills. Contacting the local community college, high school, college, or university foreign language departments may help identify individuals available as interpreters on a full- or part-time basis. Local health and social service agencies as well as the court system also may be a resource for the names of available interpreters.

What Should I Do if There Is No Trained Interpreter Available?

Several alternatives may be available for clinicians without access to a trained interpreter. Community volunteers may be a resource. Local hospitals often maintain a roster of volunteer interpreters in the community. However, health care professionals should inquire as to the qualifications of volunteer interpreters and should provide orientation as to the scope of their practice and confidentiality of patient information.

Telephone interpreter services may be an option. These services may be available within your state or locality. Throughout the country, the AT&T Language Line, 800/874-9426, is an interpreter service available in Spanish and many other languages.

Remote-simultaneous interpretation service is currently under investigation for hospitals and large clinics. This service uses patient and clinician headsets linked to a remote site to provide interpretation when an interpreter is not physically present. When evaluated, patients and physicians preferred the device to proximate-consecutive interpreter services.[9]

I Have Never Worked With an Interpreter. Is There Anything Special I Need to Do?

Physicians experienced in working with interpreters find the following recommendations helpful:

- Prior to the patient interview, discuss with the interpreter the type of interpreting you prefer.
  - Consecutive interpretation is done during a pause after each sentence or phrase. This is the most recommended method of interpreting in the clinical setting.
  - Simultaneous interpretation follows a few seconds behind as speaking continues. This type of interpretation requires an extremely high level of interpretive skills and may be too rapid and confusing for patients.
  - Summary interpretation summarizes longer blocks of information and is considered the least accurate style of interpretation.

- Ask the interpreter to introduce everyone present during the interview and explain to the patient or parent how the interpreted interview will be conducted.

- Some patients with limited English proficiency may prefer to try to speak to the physician in English, but it still is appropriate to have an interpreter present in case there are any difficulties.

- Ask the interpreter to advise you if there is anything said that he or she does not understand or is unsure how to translate so that you can rephrase the question or information.

- Allow extra time for the interview. Interpreting makes the interview take longer.

- Arrange the interview setting so that the interpreter is beside or slightly behind the patient or parent so that you maintain eye contact with the patient or parent.

- Speak directly to the patient or parent, not to the interpreter.

- Have the patient or parent repeat the instructions to ensure that your instructions were accurately interpreted.

Educational Structures in Countries of Origin

Migrant and seasonal farmworker families often emigrate from countries where the structure of education differs from that of the United States. Mexico can be used as an example to compare and contrast such differences in structures of public education systems.

Throughout Mexican history, education has been a powerful agent for social change. Mexico has one of the greatest educational traditions in the Americas. It was Mexico that opened the first university, arts academy, and public library on the North American continent.

Prior to 1988, Mexico mandated a free public education at the elementary level, providing instruction for students through the 6th grade. Students who wished to continue their education in middle school or high school had to travel to faraway cities and were required to pay for tuition and books. Poverty and a lack of transportation were some of the barriers students faced if they wished to pursue an education beyond the elementary school level. This explains why the majority of people who live in rural areas have less than a 6th grade education and why many migrant farmworkers who come to the United States from rural Mexico have low academic skills.

In 1988, President Carlos Salinas' administration reformed the national education system to include preschool and middle school in the free public education system. Now children in Mexico are required to have 1 year of prekindergarten as well as 1 year of kindergarten. This differs from the US system, where preschool and kindergarten are available options but are not required by the government. In this respect, Mexico has stronger requirements in the area of early childhood education.

In Mexico, middle school, or *secundaria,* includes grades 7, 8, and 9. Since 1988, students have been required to complete 11 years of schooling: 1 year of preschool, 1 year of kindergarten, 6 years of elementary (*primaria*), and 3 years of middle school (*secundaria*). Farmworker parents who were educated prior to 1988 often completed only 6 years of primaria.

High school is called *preparatoria,* or *bachillerato,* and includes 3 years of instruction. Education at the *preparatoria* level is optional and is not nationally funded. Tuition costs and other factors, such as distance, create barriers for many poor, rural families. Many rural villages and towns have only one elementary school and no middle school or high school. Table 1-1 compares the United States and Mexico from preschool (prekindergarten) through high school (*preparatoria*).

Another element of the educational system in Mexico is the distance learning program, or *tele secundaria,* which broadcasts middle school curriculum via satellite across Mexico. This program began 30 years ago to provide rural Mexican students with an opportunity to further their education. *Tele secundaria* is now offered in almost every school in Mexico as well as some school districts in the United States.

Table 1-1 Differences Between United States and Mexico Education Systems		
	USA Grade Level	Mexico Grade Level
Kindergarten	1	1 pre-KG
		2 KG
Elementary/*Primaria*	1	1
	2	2
	3	3
	4	4
	5	5
	6	6
Middle School/*Secundaria*	7	1
	8	2
		3*
High School/*Preparatoria* or *Bachillerato*	9	1
	10	2
	11	3
	12	

Note: In Mexico, education is only required to the secundaria level (9th-grade US system).

As a way to increase international collaboration, Mexico is currently involved in the Binational Migrant Education Program, USA-Mexico. The goal of this program is to provide continuous education to migrant students attending schools in both countries. The program ensures correct grade-age placement, transference of course credit, and school enrollment opportunities. *(See Resources.)*

References

1. US President's Commission on Migratory Labor. *Migratory Labor in American Agriculture: Report of the President's Commission on Migratory Labor.* Washington, DC: US Government Printing Office; 1951

2. Mines R, Gabbard S, Samardick R. *US Farmworkers in the Post-IRCA Period: Based on Data From the National Agricultural Workers Survey (NAWS).* Washington, DC: US Department of Labor, Office of Program Economics; 1993. (Research Report 4).

3. Miller CA, Fine A, Adams-Taylor S. *Monitoring Children's Health: Key Indicators.* 2nd ed. Washington, DC: American Public Health Association; 1989

4. American Academy of Pediatrics Task Force on Breastfeeding. Breastfeeding and the use of human milk. *Pediatrics.* 1997;100:1035-1039

5. McVea KL. Lay injection practices among migrant farmworkers in the age of AIDS: evolution of a biomedical folk practice. *Soc Sci Med.* 1997;45:91-98

6. Hatton DC. Information transmission in bilingual, bicultural contexts. *Community Health Nurs.* 1992;9:53-59

7. Brooks TR. Pitfalls in communication with Hispanic and African-American patients: do translators help or harm? *National Med Assoc.* 1992;84:941-947

8. Jacobs B. The hazards of using a child as an interpreter. *J R Soc Med.* 1995;88:474P-475P

9. Hornburger JC, Gibson CD Jr, Wood W, et al. Eliminating language barriers for non-English-speaking patients. *Med Care.* 1996;34:845-856

10. Poss JE. Working effectively with interpreters in the primary care setting. *Nurse Pract.* 1995;20:43-47

11. Prince D. Teaching Spanish to emergency medicine residents. *Acad Emerg Med.* 1995;2:32-36: discussion 36-37

Resources

Background
National Council of La Raza
1111 19th St NW, #1000
Washington, DC 20036
Telephone: 202/785-1670
Web site: http://www.nclr.org

Understanding the Cultural Context

Giblin PT. Effective utilization and evaluation of indigenous
health care workers. Review. *Public Health Rep.*
1989;104;361-68

Richter RW, Bengen B, Alsup PA, et al. The community health
worker: a resource for improved health delivery. *AJPH.*
1974;64:1056-1061

Watkins E, Larson K, Harlan C, et al. The community health
worker: a strategy for health promotion, a program evaluation, final report. *Community Health Worker.* Raleigh, NC.
1975

Wingert WA, Grubbs R, Lenoski EF, Friedman DB.
Effectiveness and efficiency of indigenous health aides in a
pediatric outpatient department. *AJPH.* 1975;65:849-857

**American Academy of Pediatrics Breastfeeding
Promotion in Pediatric Office Practices Program**
141 Northwest Point Blvd
Elk Grove Village, IL 60007
Telephone: 847/434-4000, ext 4779
Web site: http://www.aap.org

This program provides pediatricians with the latest scientific
information on breastfeeding and its management, promo-
tional materials, and strategies for increasing breastfeeding
rates in their practices.

"Call Our Pharmacist"
Telephone: 800/522-5225 or 900/903-7847

This is a for-profit hotline helping to identify foreign drugs for a fee.

Community Access to Child Health (CATCH)
Planning Funds
American Academy of Pediatrics Division of Community-based
   Initiatives
141 Northwest Point Blvd
Elk Grove Village, IL 60007-1098
Telephone: 847/434-4000, ext 4903
E-mail: catch@aap.org
Web site: http://www.aap.org

Provides grants in amounts from $2,500 to $10,000 for pediatricians and pediatric residents to hold community planning meetings, conduct needs assessment, or develop proposals for innovative, community-based child health projects

La Leche League International
1400 N Meacham Rd
PO Box 4079
Schaumburg, IL 60173-4048
Telephone: 847/519-7730 or 800/LALECHE

Provides information on breastfeeding, including educational books, brochures, and videos

National Center for Farmworker Health, Inc
PO Box 150009
Austin, TX 78715
Telephone: 512/312-2700 or 800/531-5120
Fax: 512/312-2600
Web site: http://www.ncfh.org

Provides a resource guide for lay health programs

National Center for Farmworkers Health Resource Center

1515 Capital of Texas Hwy S, Suite 220

Austin, TX 78746

Telephone: 512/328-7683

>The Diccionario de Especialidades Farmacéuticas is available through the center.

National Alliance for Hispanic Health

1501 Sixteenth St NW

Washington, DC 20036

Telephone: 202/387-5000

Fax: 202/797-4353

E-mail: publications@hispanichealth.org

>Provides the manual *Delivering Preventative Health Care to Hispanics: A Manual for Providers*. This manual provides state-of-the-art strategies for preventative health care delivery to Hispanic clients.

Pharmaceutical Research and Manufacturers Foundation of America

1100 Fifteenth St NW

Washington, DC 20005

Telephone: 202/835-3470

>Write or call for information about supplies of chronic medicines for children in financial need.

Bilingual Interpreters in the Clinical Setting

AT&T Language Line

Telephone: 800/874-9426

>Provides interpreter services in Spanish and many other languages

Educational Structures in Countries of Origin

Secretaría de Educación Pública de México. *The Modernization of Mexican Education.* [Brochure] Mexico: Secretaría de Educación Pública de México.

Secretaría de Educación Pública de México. *Normas de Inscripción, Reinscripción, Acreditación, Regularización y Certificación para Escuelas Secundarias Oficiales y Particulares Incorporadas al Sistema Educativo Nacional Período Escolar* 1996-1997. (Aug) 1996. Mexico: Secretaría de Educación Pública de México.

Binational Migrant Education Program USA-Mexico
Frank Contreras, Division of Migrant Education
Texas Education Agency
1701 N Congress Ave
Austin, TX 78701
Telephone: 512/463-9067

Chapter 2: Health Care Guidelines

Well-Child Visits

Background

Although children of migrant farmworkers have special health care concerns, they also benefit from the same basic health maintenance and anticipatory guidance as non-farmworker children. Farmworker children can and should receive a well-child examination in the same manner as any other child seen in the medical practice. Their special concerns center around the inherent risks of their lifestyle, which may parallel that of refugee children. The examining physician must keep in mind that he or she may be the only physician to ever have reviewed a particular child's health status in a comprehensive visit. Well-child examinations are an opportunity to review and examine the child with the family present and to positively impact the child's health. This process also can establish a valuable Medical Home[1] (or one of many medical homes) where the family is comfortable, the child is known, and the child's records are available.

Registration

A courteous and friendly welcome at the front desk during the registration process will greatly facilitate the pediatrician's task. Assist office staff with acquiring cross-cultural understanding and communication skills. Billing information should be obtained with a discreet and personal approach, as farmworker families often worry about the bill. These children may qualify for the Medicaid program, which provides health maintenance for low-income families. A formal chart should be made with all the necessary sections, including: a basic history questionnaire, a growth chart, and an immunization record. Age-appropriate health maintenance guidelines, like *Guidelines for Health Supervision III*, are valuable references. *(See Resources.)*

Medical History

A basic pediatric history can be obtained by a staff health worker and recorded on a standard health history form. Areas of parental concern commonly include headaches, allergies, stomachaches, perceived poor appetite, and leg aches. Such concerns may herald the diagnosis of a significant problem or they may represent a benign condition of childhood. Some parental concerns are culturally based and represent serious apprehension on the part of the parent. An example is the Mexican term *asustado,* used to describe a child that is "scared to death," or gravely ill. Ask the parent about their level of concern. It is not necessary to understand all folk illnesses if one is adept at asking questions and listening carefully. *(See Understanding the Cultural Context in Chapter 1.)*

Complete and detailed histories are sometimes difficult to elicit. For areas of the health history that are identified as serious or significant, old records can be requested from other US clinics by asking the family to sign a standard "Release of Information Form." Prior measurements of height, weight, and head circumference, as well as access to previous laboratory test results, imaging reports, and any special testing (electroencephalograms, metabolic screenings, biopsy reports, psychometric testing, etc) will greatly facilitate an accurate evaluation. Asking families ahead of time to bring all of the child's regular medicines and any available old records or addresses of previous medical providers will help. Growth and development can be assessed using a standard growth chart and a Denver Developmental test or other appropriate screening tests.

A review of systems should include assessment of

- Vision and hearing problems
- Chronic dental disease
- Chronic or recurrent infections (eg, otitis media, pneumonia, urinary tract infections, skin infections, malaria)
- Recurrent symptoms of asthma, eczema, or allergic rhinitis

- Risk of intestinal parasites (eg, chronic abdominal pain, bloating, diarrhea, poor weight gain, history of intestinal parasites in siblings or household contacts)
- Neuromuscular disabilities or seizure disorders
- Parental awareness of sexual maturation
- Behavioral concerns
- Signs of abuse or neglect

Health History Areas of High Yield

- Prenatal/perinatal history
- Growth measurements
- Diet history
- Developmental milestones
- Immunizations *(See Immunizations section.)*
- Prior hospitalizations, surgeries, injuries
- Familial diseases or premature deaths
- History of Bacille-Calmette-Guerin (BCG) vaccination, tuberculosis exposure/disease/treatment in child or family/contacts
- Exposure to environmental hazards such as pesticides, other chemicals, lead, farm machinery, home hazards *(See Environmental Concerns section.)*
- Daily mode of transportation (eg, use of car seats, pickup trucks, tractors)
- Use of home therapies, folk medicines, or imported medications
- Use of other health care providers (lay and professional)

Social History Areas of High Yield

- Family constellation
- Frequency of moves
- Type of dwelling
- Years in migrant work
- Years in the United States
- Frequency of foreign travel
- Exposure to passive smoke
- Exposure to domestic violence and firearms
- Use of child passenger safety restraints
- Learning disabilities or special needs
- Career plans (for adolescents and parents)
- Child labor history
- Family literacy level
- Need for interpreter
- School progress

Physical Examination

The circumstances of the examination should include privacy, comfort, confidentiality, and contemporary pediatric equipment as would be appreciated by any child and family in any practice.

Examinations may reveal the following:

- **Skin** often shows acute or chronic lesions such as seborrhea, eczema, scabies, pediculosis, pyoderma, acne, tinea corporis, vitiligo, or old burn injuries. A "Mongolian" hyperpigmented spot over the back and sacrum is common.

- **Ear** problems (primarily chronic and acute otitis media) are very common. Unfortunately, appropriate follow-up to ensure resolution is often difficult. Chronic middle-ear effusion with hearing loss is a frequent complication. The quality of the child's speech and/or verbal skills may be abnormal. Many children with middle-ear effusion will require regular follow-up, sometimes with prophylactic antibiotics or consultation with an otolaryngologist for possible myringotomy tube placement. A hearing screening should be conducted.

- The **eye** examination represents an opportunity to identify problems in a timely manner and avoid residual amblyopia and visual disability in the future. Common problems identified include nasolacrimal duct obstruction, conjunctivitis, corneal abrasion, strabismus, and refractive error. The necessary referral to a pediatric eye care professional and the cost of corrective lenses are frequent barriers to optimal visual acuity.

- **Dental disease** is the most common organic disease found in farmworkers and their children. *(See Oral Health section.)*

- A **cardiovascular** examination may reveal findings or defects, of which the family is unaware. Many of these children have never had a full physical examination. Normal heart sounds should be verified and any murmurs should be described in the chart. Blood pressure and femoral pulses should be checked and any signs of cyanosis, congestive heart failure, congenital heart disease, or acquired heart problems (eg, myocarditis or rheumatic valvular disease) should be noted with further investigation to follow.

- A **pulmonary** examination may show evidence of acute infection, bronchospasm, or chronic recurrent asthma. Chronic/recurrent sinusitis is common in farmworker children. Crowded home conditions and attendance at larger child care programs may be factors in the frequency of their diseases. Many children who work in the fields react to inhaled allergens and irritants. Active tuberculosis (TB) or TB disease in the pulmonary system is usually silent, identified by a positive purified protein derivative (PPD). *(See Infectious Diseases section.)*

- The **abdomen** should be carefully examined for signs of abdominal mass or hepatosplenomegaly. These children are at increased risk for enteric infections and hepatitis. These diseases can involve multiple members of the family.

- The **neck, back, and extremities** should be examined for cervical adenopathy, scoliosis, hip diseases, unequal leg length, congenital or acquired deformities, muscle atrophy, and scars from old injuries.

- A **neurologic** screening may show signs of undiagnosed cerebral palsy, or muscular or neurologic deficits. Such positive findings require a focused return visit.

- **Genitalia and Tanner Staging** need to be evaluated and documented in the examination record. Boys may have undiagnosed genital anomalies or undescended testicles. For school-age girls who are often very anxious about this part of the examination, having a parent present may be helpful. Occasionally, a female examiner can more easily complete this part of the physical examination. Care and hygiene of the male foreskin, and perineal hygiene for females, are important educational issues for disease prevention. Anticipatory guidance about sexual maturation and prevention of sexually transmitted diseases and pregnancy are needed.

Common Findings in Growth and Development Assessment

- **Short stature** is a frequent finding in farmworker children of Mexican heritage. Although usually familial, it may have other etiologies.

- **Excessive weight for height** is common and usually due to poor diet choices, over-feeding, and sedentary habits such as watching television for long periods of time. Some families have constitutionally stocky builds, and some variation should be allowed for these children as long as they are otherwise healthy and active.

- **Decreased weight for height** also is common. It may be related to several factors, including poor diet, chronic illness, or intestinal parasites. Many infants are eligible for nutrition assistance programs such as the Special Supplemental Nutrition Program for Women, Infants, and Children (WIC). Children not enrolled in nutrition assistance programs need careful review.

- **"Soft delays" in development,** particularly in language skills or fine motor function, are common as well. The family's struggle for survival may limit the amount of developmental stimulation a child may receive. Such soft delays can represent the effects of poverty, or they can be true indicators of serious developmental problems. Early involvement of the child in educationally stimulating programs followed by serial developmental assessments should clarify the child's status over time.

Laboratory Screenings

Age-appropriate laboratory screenings should be ordered according to AAP recommendations. *(See Resources.)* Special laboratory investigations and imaging procedures can be requested, as indicated by the health history and physical findings. Examples of special requests may include urinalysis, stool examination for ova and parasites, blood lead level, screenings for sexually transmitted diseases, or chest roentgenogram. Focused laboratory requests for identified risks, such as unusual infections (eg, amebiasis, cysticercosis, malaria), toxic exposures, genetic syndromes, and metabolic/endocrine diseases should be ordered as indicated. Keep in mind that the lifestyle of migrant farmworkers often limits return visits and that lab studies must include a plan for follow-up and communication with the family.

Assessment and Health Care Plan

Review all findings with the parents, and develop a health care plan addressing significant findings and future needs. Schedule follow-up appointments and necessary consultations or referrals. The plan also may address the need for case management and special services. Communication with other agencies or organizations (eg, school districts, child care programs, health departments) will facilitate a coordinated health care plan. Be mindful of parental literacy level when providing written information.

Provide a portable medical record to the family that includes your practice address, the child's acute and chronic health condition, immunization data, and all lab data, including hematocrit and TB testing. This will better protect the child and the community, as well as facilitate entry of the child into a child care program or school. Provide the family with a return appointment date and time, printed on a professional business card. Make every effort to establish an ongoing medical home for the family. Provide information on how to access care for acute illnesses or emergencies after office hours.

School Readiness

Background

School readiness is an area of concern for all children, but even more so for migrant children. Developmental delays, hearing or vision impairments, emotional difficulties, and learning problems often result from unmet health needs. Concentration is diminished when children are tired, hungry, uncomfortable, or under stress due to new surroundings and frequent moves. In addition, high rates of poverty and the lack of easy access to cultural institutions and recreation tend to trap migrant families in a world of isolation that does not adequately prepare children to enter a school setting.[2]

Approximately one third of all migrant children who do attend kindergarten are either retained or placed in a transition class instead of being promoted to first grade. The consequences of such treatment, even though often well-intentioned, are clearly detrimental. Children who stay in kindergarten an extra year are more likely to have lower self-esteem and poorer attitudes toward school.[3] A further problem is that migrant children are often placed in low-ability or remedial tracks even though they only may be limited in English language proficiency.

If migrant children are to be ready to learn when they enter school, they need opportunities to participate in early childhood education and child care programs that are developmentally, culturally, and linguistically appropriate.

History

Ask parents about the type of work they do, where they have lived, and where they have received health care. Many migrant families move several times in any given year. It also may be helpful to note the length of time parents have worked as migrant farmworkers. (Be sure to demonstrate sensitivity and confidentiality toward issues surrounding residency status.)

The parents' level of education should be determined. Immigrant parents may have had very limited opportunities to receive formal education in their native country. Ask parents about the types of programs in which a child has been enrolled. A history of participation in Early Intervention or other special education programs indicates the child has special needs that may require referral or follow up.

Because of frequent moves, many migrant children do not have access to quality preschool programs; however, frequent moves and adversity can foster resiliency. Children who migrate with their families face a variety of experiences. Along with life experiences, a child's native language should be valued as an additional special skill.

Physical Examination

In addition to the usual assessment of physical traits (height, weight, etc), gross and fine motor traits, expressive and receptive language, and personal/social traits, it also is important to note any specific observations related to a migratory lifestyle. To assess school readiness, observe how the child interacts with the parent and their communication style. Note the degree of eye contact, how the child deals with separation, and how well the child is able to follow instructions. Understand and encourage the child's interactive style and self-help capabilities.

Plan

A great deal of learning occurs before children begin school, and a parent is a child's first and most important teacher. Studies of individual families show that what the family does is more important to student success than family income or education.[4] Immigrant families, however, may have a different view on schools, teaching, and their own role in their children's education. There often is a belief that parents are not schoolteachers. Asking parents to be teachers may result in frustration and impatience among parents who feel inadequate to "teach." Parents can, however, be encouraged to seize the "teachable moment" to show preschool children how to plant a seed, write a letter, make a purchase, draw a picture using different shapes, solve a problem, or help others. They also can stimulate learning in their children by teaching them words for colors, songs, actions, animals, letters of the alphabet, and numbers. In this role, parents serve as facilitators promoting opportunities for learning.

When parents ask what they can do at home to help prepare their children for kindergarten, the best answer is READ, READ, and READ some more. To achieve the goal of school readiness, children need to be read to on a daily basis. If parents speak a language other than English, they should be encouraged to read in their home language. Local libraries should be encouraged to provide developmentally appropriate books for children in native languages that are used within the community. Encourage families to get library cards and to use local library services.[5]

For many migrant parents, however, literacy may be a problem. Parents who were educated in developing countries may have had limited opportunities to attend more than a few years of school, and they may not be comfortable reading and writing. This issue can be addressed by having items around the house that encourage reading. Magazines, newspapers, coloring books with or without words, and books of all kinds contribute to the reading environment. Magazines, such as those provided in waiting rooms of clinics and medical offices, can be given to families as a gift to promote literacy. Parents can make books for their children by cutting out pictures from magazines or by drawing their own books. Parents can "read" picture books with children and make up stories as they look at the pictures. The same book can be "read" over and over. Young children enjoy repetition.

Life experiences, experiential learning, and large motor coordination are areas that all parents can address. Natural experiences that take place at home, such as folding laundry, can be used as teaching opportunities. Parents can teach their children to count, identify shapes and colors, and problem solve by using everyday situations and activities. Storytelling, singing, and asking open-ended questions are everyday ways parents can stimulate their child's development.

Encourage parents to make appointments to visit kindergarten classrooms with their child. School personnel generally welcome such visits and children may feel more comfortable entering kindergarten if they know what it looks and feels like. Parents need to know that public schools are open to the community and that they should take the initiative to become familiar and get involved with their child's schooling.

Critical learning takes place in the infant and preschooler in all areas of development — social-emotional, cognitive, and physical. Parents who become active in their child's education during the early years (and are made to feel competent to help) will be more likely to continue to be actively involved when their children enter the upper grades. Teaching migrant parents how to use developmentally appropriate activities in their child's infancy and preschool years fosters success, confidence, and joy in learning, while providing a strong base for future success.[6]

Immunizations

Background

Three fourths of migrant children are delayed for immunizations by age 2, and many have an unknown status. They are at risk for over- and under-immunization because health care professionals may not have or may not understand the child's immunization record. Children born to mothers who did not obtain full prenatal care also are at increased risk for immunization delay.[7]

Missed opportunities to vaccinate are compounded when the child does not have an identified medical home and there is no tracking of the child's health care status on each visit. At times, there are missed opportunities because a parent associates vaccinations only with health departments or special clinics. Education and advocacy by the pediatrician on behalf of the migrating child are necessary to overcome all barriers to full immunization. As with all care to migrating children, mobility must be accounted for when scheduling vaccinations.

More than 90% of farmworker parents do carry an immunization record when given one by a health care professional. Special vaccinations (eg, for typhoid and hepatitis A) may be applicable for children migrating to high-risk areas. Risk of exposure to vaccine-preventable illnesses is increased by transnational migration; measles outbreaks have been reported in migrant communities, with spread in the preschool population. Note that receipt of a BCG vaccine does not preclude the health care professional from screening the child for tuberculosis with a PPD. *(See Infectious Diseases section.)*

History

Obtain an immunization record at the initial visit. This often means calling several health care professionals at distant sites. Records from other countries can be difficult to obtain if the parent has lost the portable card. In such instances, immunizations need to be started over again, although this would be a rare scenario. Occasionally, the child's prior school district may be located more easily than his or her health care professional. Immunization records may be available by telephone from school personnel.

It is helpful to become familiar with the Mexican immunization schedule. Until recently, measles vaccine (sarampión) was given without mumps and rubella combined. Presently, MMR is given to children at 12 months of age. A copy of the national Mexican immunization schedule is found in Table 2-1.

Table 2-1 Mexican Immunization Schedule			
Vacuna (Vaccine)	Enfermedad que previene (Illiness it Prevents)	Dosis (Dose)	Edad (Age)
BCG	Tuberculosis	1st	Al nacer (at birth)
Sabin	Poliomielitis (Polio)	Preliminar (Preliminary)	Al nacer
		1st	2 meses (2 months)
		2nd	4 meses (4 months)
		3rd	6 meses (6 months)
		Adicionales (Additional)	Semanas Nacionales de Vacunacion (National Vaccination Weeks)
Penta Valente (no US equivalent)	Difteria (Diphtheria) Tosferina (Pertussis) Tetanos (Tetanus) H. Influenzae b Hepatitis B	1st	2 meses
		2nd	4 meses
		3rd	6 meses
DPT	Difteria (Diphtheria) Tosferina (Pertussis) Tetanos (Tetanus)	Refuerzo (Booster)	2 años (2 years)
		Refuerzo	4 años (4 years)
Triple Viral (MMR)	Sarampión (Measles) Rubéola (Rubella) Parotiditis (Mumps)	1st	12 meses
		2nd	6 anos
TD	Tétanos Difteria	Refuerzo	12 anos

From the 1999 National Mexican Immunization Schedule found in La Cartilla Nacional de Vacunación.

Generally recognized barriers to age-appropriate immunization include the following: lack of a medical home, rural dwelling, parental education of less than 12th grade, lack of insurance, and residence in a family with two or more children. These barriers apply to most children of farmworkers. Although immunization delay in the United States has been blamed in part on parental opposition to vaccines or fear of pain and side effects, this barrier is generally not an issue for farmworker families. Ask the parents why the child has not received each vaccination on schedule, and assist the family in planning for appropriate receipt of subsequent vaccines.

Include in the history the frequency of travel (out of state and out of country). Document the child's mobility pattern and plan immunizations such that all opportunities to vaccinate are optimized. For example, if the child is departing the area in 6 weeks to an unknown destination, and will be due for a routine immunization in 2 months, have the child return to you prior to departure and use the accelerated schedule as found in the *2000 Red Book. (See Infectious Diseases section of the Resources for publication information.)* This applies as well to those children traveling to developing countries. *(See Tables 2-2 and 2-3.)*

Physical Examination

While there are no specific guidelines linking physical examinations and immunizations, it is extremely important not to isolate immunization visits from more complete child health assessments that include a thorough history and physical. Many migrant children have received fragmented health care services, often initiated by child care or school personnel, with an emphasis on immunizations, but may suffer a neglect of their general health. Conversely, some health care professionals see these children for acute care visits but do not provide immunizations apart from designated well-child visits. Children of migrant farmworkers have such barriers to regular access to care that consideration of the child's comprehensive care needs must be a part of every visit.

Table 1.5. **Recommended Immunization Schedules for Children Not Immunized in the First Year of Life***

Recommended Time/Age	Immunization(s)†	Comments
Younger Than 7 Years		
First visit	DTaP, Hib,‡ HBV, MMR	If indicated, tuberculin testing may be done at same visit. If child is 5 y of age or older, Hib is not indicated in most circumstances.
Interval after first visit		
1 mo (4 wk)	DTaP, IPV, HBV, Var§	The second dose of IPV may be given if accelerated poliomyelitis immunization is necessary, such as for travelers to areas where polio is endemic.
2 mo	DTaP, Hib,‡ IPV	Second dose of Hib is indicated only if the first dose was received when younger than 15 mo.
≥8 mo	DTaP, HBV, IPV	IPV and HBV are not given if the third doses were given earlier.
Age 4–6 y (at or before school entry)	DTaP, IPV, MMR‖	DTaP is not necessary if the fourth dose was given after the fourth birthday; IPV is not necessary if the third dose was given after the fourth birthday.
Age 11–12 y	See Fig 1.1, p 22	
7–12 Years		
First visit	HBV, MMR, dT, IPV	
Interval after first visit		
2 mo (8 wk)	HBV, MMR,‖ Var,§ dT, IPV	IPV also may be given 1 mo after the first visit if accelerated poliomyelitis immunization is necessary.
8–14 mo	HBV,¶ dT, IPV	IPV is not given if the third dose was given earlier.
Age 11–12 y	See Fig 1.1, p 22	

* Table is not completely consistent with all package inserts. For products used, also consult manufacturer's package insert for instructions on storage, handling, dosage, and administration. Biologics prepared by different manufacturers may vary, and package inserts of the same manufacturer may change. Therefore, the physician should be aware of the contents of the current package insert. Vaccine abbreviations: HBV indicates hepatitis B virus; Var, varicella; DTaP, diphtheria and tetanus toxoids and acellular pertussis; Hib, *Haemophilus influenzae* type b conjugate; IPV, inactivated poliovirus; MMR, live measles-mumps-rubella; dT, adult tetanus toxoid (full dose) and diphtheria toxoid (reduced dose), for children 7 years of age or older and adults.

Table 1.5. Recommended Immunization Schedules for
Children Not Immunized in the First Year of Life, * continued

† If all needed vaccines cannot be administered simultaneously, priority should be given to protecting the child against the diseases that pose the greatest immediate risk. In the United States, these diseases for children younger than 2 years usually are measles and *Haemophilus influenzae* type b infection; for children older than 7 years, they are measles, mumps, and rubella. Before 13 years of age, immunity against hepatitis B and varicella should be ensured. DTaP, HBV, Hib, MMR, and Var can be given simultaneously at separate sites if failure of the patient to return for future immunizations is a concern. For further information on pertussis and poliomyelitis immunization, see the respective chapters (Pertussis, p 435, and Poliovirus Infections, p 465).

‡ See *Haemophilus influenzae* Infections, p 262, and Table 3.11 (p 268).

§ Varicella vaccine can be administered to susceptible children any time after 12 months of age. Unimmunized children who lack a reliable history of varicella should be immunized before their 13th birthday.

|| Minimal interval between doses of MMR is 1 month (4 wk).

¶ HBV may be given earlier in a 0-, 2-, and 4-month schedule.

From American Academy of Pediatrics. Active and Passive Immunization. In: Pickering LK, ed. *2000 Red Book: Report of the Committee on Infectious Diseases.* 25th ed. Elk Grove Village, IL: American Academy of Pediatrics; 2000:24

Table 2-3
Recommended Immunizations for Travelers to Developing Countries*

Immunizations	Length of Travel		
	Brief, <2 wk	Intermediate, 2 wk to 3 mo	Long-term Residential, >3 mo
Review and complete age-appropriate childhood schedule (see text for details) • DTaP, poliovirus vaccine, and *Haemophilus influenzae* type b vaccine may be given at 4-wk intervals if necessary to complete the recommended schedule before departure • Measles: 2 additional doses given if younger than 12 mo of age at first dose • Varicella • Hepatitis B[†]	+	+	+
Yellow fever[‡]	+	+	+
Hepatitis A[§]	+	+	+
Typhoid fever[§]	±	+	+
Meningococcal disease[||]	±	±	±
Rabies[¶]	±	+	+
Japanese encephalitis[‡]	±	±	+

* See disease-specific chapters in Section 3 for details. For further sources of information, see text. DTaP indicates diphtheria and tetanus toxoids and acellular pertussis; +, recommended; and ±, consider.
† If insufficient time to complete 6-month primary series, accelerated series can be given (see text for details).
‡ For endemic regions *(see Health Information for International Travel*, p 3). For high-risk activities in areas experiencing outbreaks, vaccine is recommended even for brief travel.
§ Indicated for travelers who will consume food and liquids in areas of poor sanitation.
|| For endemic regions of Africa, during local epidemics, and travel to Saudi Arabia for the Hajj.
¶ Indicated for person with high risk of animal exposure, and for travelers to endemic countries.

This table is from American Academy of Pediatrics. Active and Passive Immunization. In: Pickering LK, ed. *2000 Red Book: Report of the Committee on Infectious Diseases.* 25th ed. Elk Grove Village, IL. American Academy of Pediatrics; 2000:78

It is not unusual to find appropriately immunized migrant children with unrecognized delays in development, congenital abnormalities such as heart defects, and problems made more severe by lack of an early diagnosis (such as the complete dislocation of a hip in a 2 year old).

Treatment Plan

- Avoid missing opportunities to vaccinate. Note the barriers experienced by the family in immunizing their child, and develop a plan to overcome those barriers.

- Check the child's immunization status at each office visit.

- Provide simultaneous administration of all needed vaccines rather than requiring separate visits.

- Provide each migrant family with a portable record that includes immunization information as well as your office telephone number and address.

- Use audiovisual educational materials in the waiting room, such as the video "Before It's Too Late, Vaccinate," available from the American Academy of Pediatrics in English and Spanish. *(See Resources.)*

- Conduct regular chart reviews of your migrant patients to ascertain immunization needs. Develop a tracking system for your migrant patients.

- Consider incentives for immunization such as Polaroid photos of the child or a certificate on completion of immunizations at age 2.

- Use the "catch-up" schedule, as recommended in the *2000 Red Book,* for children with immunization delays. Provide an accelerated schedule for high-risk children who may move before completing immunizations on a traditional schedule.

- Obtain information on vaccine-preventable outbreaks in foreign countries by contacting the Centers for Disease Control and Prevention 24-hour hotline, 404/332-4559.

Adolescent Care

Background

An estimated 36,000 children of migrant laborers engage in farm work.[8] About 169,000 more youth under the age of 21 travel to do farm work *without* their parents.[9] Because many of these adolescents work full time and even marry at early ages (13 to 17),[10] the traditional distinctions between early, middle, and late adolescent developmental stages may be less valid in this population. However, these adolescents, like their non-migrant peers, are undergoing significant physical and psychological changes that can lead to emotional disorders and health-risk behaviors. Although data describing adolescent morbidity in the migrant population are largely unavailable, health care professionals need to emphasize preventive services and health screening in this high-risk group.

History

Adolescents in this population should be assessed for the following:

- Respiratory and ear infections
- Bacterial and viral gastroenteritis
- Intestinal parasites
- Skin infections
- Scabies and head lice
- Pesticide exposure
- Tuberculosis
- Poor nutrition
- Anemia
- Short stature
- Intentional and unintentional injuries
- Substance abuse
- Teenage pregnancy
- Dental decay
- School absenteeism

Other issues clinicians should pay particular attention to include

- Migrant women are more likely to have **urinary tract infections** because of long workdays, no bathroom facilities, and poor hygienic conditions.[10]

- **Acne and eczema** are more likely among indigent Mexican American adolescents.[11] Exposure to fertilizers and pesticides account for many of these conditions, as do malnutrition and vitamin deficiency.

- Overcrowded living conditions lead to **lice infestation.**[12]

- **Diabetes and hypertension** are common in adults and often have their beginnings in adolescence due to diet and lifestyle patterns.[2, 12, 13]

- Working adolescents are at risk for all of the **occupational diseases** of adult farmworkers.

Women in this culture marry early and often have begun to have children when they are 13 to 17 years old, resulting in high teenage pregnancy rates. While there are insufficient data on birth outcomes of migrant teenage pregnancies, studies suggest that these individuals seek prenatal care later than acculturated teenagers,[14] and prenatal care, when sought, is often fragmented.[12] Sexually active adolescents are at risk for sexually transmitted diseases, including HIV.

There are few data regarding mental health issues among migrant adolescents. It is clear that the migrant family leads a transient and uncertain life with long, stressful hours compensated with very low wages. Lacking job security, education, transportation, health care, and social services, migrant teenagers are predisposed to domestic violence and substance abuse.

Physical Examination

The American Medical Association's *Guidelines for Adolescent Preventive Services (GAPS)* is highly relevant to migrant farmworkers' adolescent dependents and those adolescents working independently in the fields and orchards. The GAPS summarizes the preventive services and screening recommendations for this specific population.[12] From ages 11 to 21 years, all adolescents should have an annual routine health visit. Preventive services should be age appropriate, developmentally appropriate, and sensitive to individual and sociocultural differences.

The GAPS recommends a complete physical examination during three of the annual health visits between 11 and 21 years. Because of the increased number of health problems of migrant adolescents and likelihood that many annual visits will be missed, complete physical examinations are appropriate whenever the adolescent is able to keep his or her office appointment. Special attention should be paid to growth parameters, blood pressure measurements, and sexual maturity assessment.

Health Promotion

- Migrant adolescents should receive annual counseling to promote healthy diets and injury prevention.
- All adolescents should be counseled regarding responsible sexual behavior, including abstinence. Migrant teenagers should be counseled about protection from sexually transmitted diseases, including HIV, and latex condoms should be available with instruction on how to use them effectively.
- Counseling on avoidance of all tobacco products, alcohol, and drugs should be given.
- Risk for emotional problems should be assessed, including screening factors for depression and suicide.
- All adolescents should receive annual assessments of educational progress.
- The presence of physical and sexual abuse and domestic violence should be assessed.
- Occupational history should be taken and appropriate education should be given regarding risk reduction in the workplace.

Screening

Screening for hypertension should be done at each visit because adolescent farmworkers often do not regularly complete an annual physical examination. Hyperlipidemia screening should be considered for adolescents thought to be at risk for cardio-vascular disease. Sexually active males should have a screening urinalysis for leukocyte esterase for nongonococcal urethritis. Human immunodeficiency virus testing should be offered to all adolescents. Tuberculosis screening should be done annually in this high-risk population. *(See Infectious Diseases section.)*

Treatment and Special Considerations

Confidential care to migrant adolescents deserves careful consideration. The pediatric health care professional must consider the unique cultural background of Hispanic patients and understand issues concerning ethnic affiliation, family support systems, religious beliefs, customs regarding communication, and cultural beliefs concerning illness.[15] The pediatric health care professional must elicit the adolescent's perspective about his or her health issues and take a "cultural assessment."[15,16] Models have been developed to help pediatric health care professionals more effectively extract culture-specific information. *(See Resources in this chapter, and Understanding the Cultural Context in Chapter 1.)* Moreover, communication difficulties may necessitate the use of an interpreter. Family translators may be inappropriate in situations where the information sought from the adolescent is sensitive and should remain confidential. The ideal translator is culturally sensitive and independent from the family, is an advocate of the adolescent, and is able to deliver effective health counseling. Suggestions for working with translators and adolescents are available.[15,16] *(See also Bilingual Interpreters in the Clinical Setting in Chapter 1.)*

An understanding of acculturation is necessary in caring for migrant adolescents. For instance, health knowledge, health behavior, and school performance may change with the length of time the adolescent has been in the United States.[14,16] While acculturation is to some extent inevitable and important to successful integration into a new culture, adolescents who are immigrants are confronted with a unique dilemma. Confusion about acculturation interfaces with the normal developmental crisis of adolescence and heightens the struggle in socialization and identity formation.[15] Successful acculturation may directly conflict with parental expectations, which may further increase stress in the adolescent.[16]

Finally, as with care delivered to younger children, adolescent patients should be provided with a portable record describing their health problems, immunizations, medications, and treatment needs.

Oral Health

Background

Dental problems rank as the most common diagnosis for children ages 10 to 14, second most common for ages 15 to 19, and eighth most common for migrant patients of all ages.[17] The progression of early childhood caries (ECC), also called baby bottle tooth decay, may affect the child's growth adversely.[18] Studies now suggest that the same prone feeding position that causes nursing caries also increases the child's risk for otitis media.[19,20] The incidence of ECC is epidemic among children of migrant farmworkers. Numerous studies show the overall rates of dental disease are significantly higher in these children than in the average child in the United States. A 1987 report showed that only 23% of the migrant children examined in Colorado were free of dental decay.[21] Data collected in the Yakima Valley of central Washington showed that migrant children suffered from decay rates two to three times the national average.[22] Other studies from Connecticut,[23] Florida,[24] and New York[25] show a population with high dental needs and little access to care. These reports show only the amount and not the severity of disease. While disease severity is difficult to measure, a statewide survey in Washington showed that up to 18% of the low-income children had emergent dental needs, defined as children stating pain.

Barriers to Good Oral Health

Many migrant children lack access to health care.[26] Few agricultural employers offer health insurance, particularly plans with dental coverage. Even when these children are eligible for Medicaid dental services, most state programs' payments are so low that few dentists accept such coverage for payment. Those dentists who do see low-income children often are not equipped to handle the language differences. The migrant farmworker population has only a few public health dentists and private sector dentists who will offer a reduced fee or free services. As a result, dental care for migrant farmworkers often tends to be episodic and emergent in nature.

Sometimes, migrant children may not be in the area long enough for completion of care. Delivering dental care to young children is particularly difficult. These children need to trust the dental team. Frequent short visits designed to enhance the child's cooperation are ideal but rarely possible for the migrant child due to crowded dental facilities and the inability of parents to take time off from work.

The living conditions of most migrant families also may preclude proper care of the teeth. Migrant children use medical services more readily than dental services. This is especially true for children younger than 3 years of age. Preventing dental disease in this younger age group is the greatest hope we have in improving the oral health of migrant children. Physicians are experts in applying the medical model to fight infectious diseases. If this approach can be applied nationwide in fighting dental disease in the 0- to 3-year-old population, pediatricians can have a far greater impact on the oral health of not only migrant children but all low-income children. Physicians need to understand that intercepting the caries process of enamel demineralization, which begins to occur at 12 to 18 months of age (months before cavities are observed), is the key to successful preventive dentistry.

Dental Disease Patterns

The following three ingredients are needed for a tooth to decay: a tooth, cariogenic bacteria, and fermentable carbohydrates. Acquisition of cariogenic bacteria is necessary, but alone is not sufficient to promote the caries process. Salivary flow, access to fluoride, dietary habits, bacterial virulence, tooth morphology, and other factors modify the caries process. It is important to have some understanding of decay patterns to better assess, prevent, and refer for appropriate treatment. If caries/decay is identified by the physician, good home care must be stressed and the patient referred to a dentist, if possible. The four decay patterns seen in children are as follows:

- **Caries from hypoplasia.** This is decay from defects in the tooth enamel. These defects can be seen when the teeth erupt and are susceptible to decay. Often, the defects are seen at the cutting (incisal) edge of the top front teeth.

- **Occlusal (pit and fissure) caries.** This decay forms on the chewing surfaces of the teeth. Measures to prevent occlusal caries include adequate and frequent tooth brushing and dental sealants. Sealants are a plastic-like coating that can be applied to the occlusal surface of a tooth that fills in the grooves and prevents bacteria from establishing in and eventually decaying these surfaces. Sealants are applied on primary and permanent molar teeth, although few state Medicaid programs pay for primary sealants. Children can receive sealants in dental offices and through school sealant programs.

- **Smooth surface caries.** This decay can be found on the cheek (buccal) and tongue (lingual) side of the teeth and between the teeth. Preventive procedures include daily flossing to keep bacterial colonies from forming as well as fluoride from water fluoridation, applied fluoride products in the dental office, and home fluoride products.

- ECC. This is a distinctive and destructive pattern of tooth decay in the primary dentition. In its most aggressive form, it can completely destroy the crowns of the maxillary anterior teeth by the age of 18 months. In the early stages, decay or white spot lesions often can be seen in the middle of the buccal or lingual surfaces of the top front teeth or on the tooth at the gum line. Early childhood caries is caused by the introduction of Strepmutans and related bacteria into the child's mouth as teeth erupt before normal bacterial colonization of the child's mouth occurs (12 to 33 months). The source of the caries producing Strepmutans bacteria is known to be the child's mother or close caregiver. Identifying close caregivers who have active caries or broken/fractured dental restorations and helping them seek dental care before this "window of infectivity" opens (12 to 33 months) is an important part of preventing ECC. When combined with improper infant feeding practices, the infection causes severe destruction of the primary dentition, pain, and swelling. In other words, children who are put to bed and breastfeed or suck on a bottle continuously, without detaching throughout the night, are at high risk for ECC in this population because of the poor dental health of the parents. Numerous studies now show that children with ECC are at greater risk for future caries than children without ECC. Because of the extensive treatment needs and young ages often associated with ECC, hospitalization is often required, adding to the cost of this dental condition. Prevention of ECC includes oral health promotion and education, for the parent as well as for the child. A well-organized medical oral health promotion/education campaign combined with a regimented dental project using applied chemotherapeutic agents, such as chlorhexadine mouth rinses for the parent and fluoride varnish for the child, may prove to be a powerful preventive approach to this costly and devastating dental problem.

Recognition of the basic decay patterns is indicative of the child's past and future caries experience and may help to determine preventive and referral measures. Caries patterns are critical in identifying children whose disease can be prevented, and prevention is the area where medical professionals can have a dramatic impact on the oral health of this population.

Dental Examination in the Medical Clinic

All children should receive a dental examination during a medical physical examination. This is of critical importance for children of migrant farmworkers because the likelihood of accessing a dentist is low. Instruments needed for a dental examination are gauze, a tongue blade, and a good light source. Dental examinations from birth to age $2\frac{1}{2}$ are best done in the lap position. The parent holds the child and places the child's head in the lap of the physician. This way the parent is able to control the child during the procedure. You may need to wipe the teeth clean with gauze before the quick assessment can be done. Oral assessments on older children can be done with the child sitting with his or her head tipped slightly backward. A dental mirror is useful for these examinations, but is not necessary.

When examining the dentition of infants and toddlers, look particularly at the cheek and tongue sides of the top anterior teeth for cavitated lesions or "white spots." The type of spots that signify pathology will appear as chalky white, soft-appearing areas either at the gingival line or in the center of the tooth. Often, they are found when the tooth is wiped free of plaque. Infants and toddlers with white spot lesions and a positive history of improper feeding practices should be the focus of dental disease prevention. **Early identification of demineralized enamel before cavitation occurs (white spots), combined with topical fluorides, improved oral hygiene, and appropriate feeding habits, frequently leads to remineralization of the damaged enamel and eliminates the need for restorative dental care.**

Assessment

Once cavitation of enamel has occurred, treatment in the medical office is rather limited. If purulent infection is present, antibiotics and pain medication will relieve the acute problem, but the patient requires a dental referral for the surgical repair or extraction of the tooth. The same is true when assessing children who have no pain but obvious decay. Because referral sources will most likely be limited, assessing patients who already have dental disease, while important, will produce only limited health improvement for the migrant community in general. Assessment for disease prevention, however, will produce significant results and should be based on the dental health history provided by the child's primary caregiver.

Oral Health Promotion and Education

Oral health education should be age and risk appropriate as well as a standard part of prenatal health promotion. Children are not born with oral bacteria. They generally acquire this flora from their primary caretaker through simple child care activities like kissing or blowing on or pretesting food. A large and early transfer of caries-producing bacteria combined with poor nutritional practices, such as nighttime bottle feeding, can have a devastating effect on a toddlers' dentition.

- Look in the mouths of your pregnant patients and impress on them the need for basic dental home care practices not only for their health but also for the health of their babies.

- Teach parents to use the bottle only while cradling their child and never to allow their child to fall asleep with the bottle in their mouths.

- Explain to the breastfeeding mother that breast milk, like other foods, can promote tooth decay if the baby has weak enamel. Like all parents, she needs to pay close attention to oral hygiene.

- Encourage moms to wean the toddler off the bottle by age 1. Concentrate on the positive message of encouraging the use of "no-spill" or "tippy" cups instead of admonishing parents about the nighttime bottle habit. Discourage parents from using the cups "on demand" for juice and other sugary products.

- Teach parents the simple technique of lifting the child's lip and looking at the teeth on a regular basis and to be on guard for developing changes in the appearance of the teeth, like chalky white spots.

- Instruct parents to clean the baby's teeth at least twice a day, in the morning and before bedtime. Parents may want to begin by wiping the teeth with a clean soft washcloth, but should introduce a toothbrush before 12 months of age and use small amounts of toothpaste. Only small amounts of a fluoride toothpaste ($\frac{1}{4}$ to $\frac{1}{2}$ pea-size amount) are necessary to provide the child an anticariogenic benefit. Excessive amounts of swallowed fluoride toothpaste can lead to dental fluorosis of the permanent teeth, but this is not a common problem in this population of children that has such a high caries rate.

- As the child gets older and as the parent's dental awareness grows, introduce daily flossing. Parents should be encouraged to brush and floss their child's teeth until the child is proficient, usually about 6 years of age.

Bleeding gums (gingivae) in children is an early warning sign that proper home care is not being practiced. Generally, it can be treated with proper brushing. Advise using a soft bristle brush and have the parent gently brush the gums and teeth. Demonstrate this technique to the parent. If proper oral hygiene is done in the home, bleeding gums should clear up in about a week. Bleeding gingivae also can be a sign of an underlying systemic disease. If good home care does not alleviate the bleeding, a more thorough medical examination is indicated.

Take a common sense, non-blaming approach and do not overload the parent with information. Concentrate on the biggest problem you see. If the teeth are caked with plaque, concentrate on brushing. If the infant has white spot lesions on the top, front teeth, take the time to discover what is going on in the home.

Preventive Treatments

Currently there only are a few preventive products available for use to fight dental disease in children.

- **Fluoride supplements:** For children whose known water source contains inadequate fluoride levels, prescriptions for flouride supplements should be a mainstay of any preventive dental program. Fluoride is best prescribed only if the fluoride content is known. If risk assessment for caries is high and the child's primary water source cannot be identified, however, prescribing supplemental fluoride is appropriate.

This information can be very difficult to obtain for migrant children living in rural areas. Table 2-4 shows the current fluoride supplement prescribing protocols.[27] Many school programs give out fluoride prescriptions. Call your local schools and inquire if they have an active fluoride prescription program.

- **Fluoride varnish:** While new to this country, fluoride varnish has been used in Europe for 20 years as an effective decay-preventive agent. Simply put, it is a high concentration of fluoride in a viscous varnish medium that can be painted, in small amounts, on the teeth of children at specific time intervals. Numerous studies have shown that it yields comparable results to the more familiar tray fluoride treatments given in dental offices, yet it is easier and safer to use in very young children.[28] To apply fluoride varnish, wipe the teeth dry with gauze and apply the varnish with a disposable brush. Generally, less than 0.3 mL of varnish is required to paint all the primary teeth. When used in conjunction with other health promotion activities, it can be a very effective public health approach to preventing dental disease in immigrant and other low-income populations with poor access to dental care. Currently, its use is slowly gaining acceptance in community/migrant health center dental programs. To date, there are no studies using fluoride varnish outside of individ-

Table 2-4 Fluoride Supplement Prescribing Protocols			
Age	Concentration of Fluoride in Drinking Water		
	Less than 0.3 ppm	0.3 to 0.6 ppm	More than 0.6 ppm
6 months to 3 years	0.25 mg	0 mg	0 mg
3 to 6 years	0.5 mg	0.25 mg	0 mg
6 to 16 years	1.00 mg	0.5 mg	0 mg

ppm = parts per million

ually designed preventive programs in a dental office and, therefore, there are no established protocols for use in a public health arena.

- **Xylitol gum:** Research is showing that xylitol can be a very effective decay-preventive agent. To achieve good results, xylitol gum needs to be chewed for at least 5 minutes, twice a day.[29] Xylitol gum can be difficult for patients to find, but keep this product in mind for your gum-chewing patients.

Referrals

While the medical profession can be an extremely effective force in oral health promotion, you will encounter children in need of treatment. Dental referral sources will vary from region to region, but most likely they will be limited. If so, you need to determine the child's risk through assessment and triage and refer according to your referral availability. Dental disease in the migrant population is not just a dental problem; it is an overall health concern. Involve your medical and dental community to develop ways to encourage and open up the referral system.

Nutritional Status

Background

Few studies relate specifically to the nutritional status and dietary habits of farmworker children. However, because farmworker children are among the poorest children in the United States and many migrant farmworker families are recent immigrants, the nutritional risks associated with poverty and minority status apply to these children. Migrant farmworker children's nutritional status may be particularly at risk because of the disruption to the household due to frequent moves and the extremely poor housing available to migrant families.

Dairy foods are the main source of calcium for Mexican Americans; however, corn tortillas also are an important source of calcium in their diet.[30] Traditional Mexican diets offer protective benefits when compared with the typical US diet. These benefits disappear as acculturation increases.[31] Fat consumption increases among Hispanics as they become acculturated in the United States.[32]

Lack of access to refrigeration and clean water make bottle-feeding particularly dangerous for the migrant child. Continued breastfeeding offers considerable immunological as well as nutritional benefits for the migrant child.[33] Early discontinuation of breastfeeding is common among Mexican women. The mean age for weaning is 4 months.[34] The introduction of juice and solids by 3 months is common in low-income Mexican populations.[35]

Migrant farmworkers may have little knowledge about the relationship between food consumption and health.[36] Additionally, the need for exercise may not be well understood. A study of girls in grades 5 through 12 found that the Hispanic group reported lower activity levels than other racial groups. Only 36% met the Year 2000 goal for strenuous activity.[37]

History

Interview to obtain the following information:

Social History

- Identify the primary caregiver of the child and others assisting in feeding. Is there a grandmother in the home assisting with the child's care?

- Does the child attend a child care center, Head Start, school?

- Elicit parent/caregiver's concerns regarding the child's appetite, eating habits, health, and growth. How do the parents regard obesity in children? Is it seen as a sign of health, offering protection during illness? Are there concerns about lifelong health consequences of obesity?

- Ask for information on the family's food purchasing, storage, and preparation resources. Does the family have access to a refrigerator and/or stove?

- Is the child enrolled in the WIC and/or food stamp program?

Dietary History

- Elicit the parent/caregiver's perception of an appropriate diet for the child.

- Ask the parent/caregiver to recall the amount and types of food consumed by the child in the last 24 hours. Ask about food frequency (food groups and key nutrient foods consumed during past week).

- Does the child have food allergies or intolerances? Does the child refuse certain foods or types of food?

- Which ethnic foods are consumed? What is the degree of acculturation to US eating patterns?

- For infants, what is the frequency and duration of breast-feeding and what is the type and amount of formula used, method of formula preparation, and use of pacifier and bedtime bottle?

- Have the parent/caregiver describe the general appetite, digestive complaints, and bowel habits.

- What is the water source? Is water fluoridated at home and school? *(See Oral Health section.)*

- What is the use of vitamin supplements, herbs, or special foods for health?

- Does the child ingest nonfood items (pica)?

- What is the child's activity level? Is there access to safe play areas?

Familial Risk Factors

- Is there a family history of obesity, diabetes, or hypertension?

Physical Examination

Mexican American farmworker children and adolescents are consistently found to be at increased risk for obesity. Based on evaluations of infants and preschoolers, 18% were at or above the 90th percentile for weight-for-length or height.[38] The prevalence of obesity has increased over time in Mexican American children and youth.[39,40] Among Hispanic school-aged children, the body mass index was strongly correlated with increased risk for hypertension. This confirms that overweight children are significantly more likely to have elevated systolic blood pressures and total blood cholesterol levels, and that weight reduction may play an important role in reducing coronary heart disease in this population.[41]

A study of migrant children in North Carolina found that short stature among Mexican American children is common. Ten percent of preschoolers fall below the 5th percentile for height-for-age.[38] Another study of young children in Mexico found that short stature is common and that growth stunting is thought to occur in Mexican children during early infancy.[42]

The diets of migrant preschool children have been found to be deficient in recommended servings of fruits and vegetables, and only one fourth of the children in one study had the recommended three servings from the milk group. Adequate protein did not appear to be a problem. Almost all met or exceeded the recommended daily allowance for protein.[38]

Assessment should cover the following areas:

Anthropometric

- Record height, weight, and growth percentiles.
- Evaluate whether height and weight are appropriate for age.
- Determine if weight is appropriate for length or height.
- Evaluate for "failure to thrive" and any inappropriate changes in growth patterns if prior growth information is available.

Clinical

- Take blood pressure for children 2 years of age and older.
- Examine skin, hair, and nails for signs of nutrient deficiencies.
- Assess clinical signs of nutrient deficiencies; perform further tests as indicated.
- Assess dental status — appearance of decay, nursing bottle syndrome, gum disease, poor dental hygiene, and impact of dental status on dietary intake. *(See Oral Health section.)*
- Determine fluoride intake from all sources.
- Determine if presence of parasitic infection is compromising nutritional status.

Dietary

- Evaluate dietary intake for energy and nutrient requirements, including protein, iron, and vitamins A and C.
- Assess dietary intake of sodium, saturated fat, cholesterol, and sugar.
- Evaluate impact of feeding practices on child's dietary intake and health.
- Determine the safety of water source. *(See Groundwater Contamination section.)*

Social

- Assess caregiver's knowledge of an appropriate diet for the child and the need for nutritional education and assistance with meal planning.

- Assess family's resources to purchase and prepare adequate diet.

Laboratory Screenings

Latin American immigrants are at increased risk and should be screened for iron-deficiency anemia, intestinal parasites, and dental problems.[43] Iron deficiency rates are higher among low-income and Hispanic children, which means that Mexican American migrant children are especially at risk.[44] Conduct hemoglobin and hematocrit tests to screen for iron deficiency anemia. Evaluate blood work for iron-deficiency anemia and plumbism and order further tests as needed. Examine stool for ova, giardia antigen, and parasites.

Assessment and Plan

Physician recommendations can have an impact on family nutritional behaviors. Family-oriented nutritional counseling of obese Mexican Americans, that also is culturally and linguistically appropriate, can achieve significant weight reduction in this population.[45] Discussion of family opportunities for recreational exercise (such as walking, soccer, frisbee) also can be helpful.

It is essential that health care professionals be supportive of the mother's intention to breastfeed and supportive of continued breastfeeding. The advice to breastfeed from prenatal care and WIC professionals is the strongest predictor of breastfeeding among Mexican American women.[46]

Guidance to the parents should address the following areas:

Anthropometric

- Discuss child's growth and weight assessment and any significant risk factors, such as obesity.

Clinical

- Discuss assessment findings and any nutritional risk factors.
- Prescribe fluoride supplements and/or treatments as indicated.
- Review the availability of electricity, safe drinking water, and food storage capacities.
- Discuss the means for hand washing and utensil cleaning in food preparation.
- Refer for dental services when appropriate.
- Prescribe vitamin/mineral supplements as needed.
- Arrange for follow-up or referral as needed for any problems identified.

Dietary

- Encourage continued breastfeeding and provide information on the health benefits of breastfeeding.
- Discuss appropriate infant feeding practices to avoid ECC. *(See Oral Health section.)* Discuss recommended changes in feeding practices. Encourage weaning from bottle to cup by 1 year of age.
- Discuss dietary risk factors based on 24-hour recall and food frequency. Discuss recommended changes in quality and/or quantity of diet. Provide an example of a daily meal plan and serving sizes for the child using low-cost foods familiar to the family.
- Encourage increased intake of foods rich in iron, vitamin A, and calcium. Provide examples of foods familiar to the family that are low in cost and high in these nutrients.

- Caution parents about excessive use of high-sugar, high-fat, nutrient-poor foods. Discuss appropriate snacks with consideration as to cost, practicality, and ethnic food preferences of the family.

- Counsel female teenagers about foods high in folic acid and the importance of preconception health when appropriate. Recommend vitamin supplementation to ensure folic acid intake.

- Enlist the help of a nutritionist to guide you in the preparation of these recommendations.

- Discuss use of any dietary practices used as home remedies.

Social

- Refer to WIC and/or food stamps or other food assistance programs if appropriate.

- Counsel parents about appropriate precautions to ensure safe water supply for drinking and formula preparation.

- Recommend appropriate physical exercise and activities.

Environmental Concerns

Lead Poisoning

Background

Lead poisoning is the most common disease of toxic environmental origin among children in the United States today.[47] The Centers for Disease Control and Prevention (CDC) estimates that 930,000 children aged 1 to 5 years currently have blood lead levels of 10 µg/dL or greater.[48]

Blood lead levels in the United States have declined dramatically over the past 2 decades; from 1976 to 1994 the prevalence of blood lead levels greater than 10 µg/dL decreased by 94%.[48] This decline principally is due to removal of lead from gasoline and, additionally, to bans on the use of lead in household paint, food and drink cans, and plumbing systems.[49]

Despite the decline in blood lead levels, the risk of lead exposure remains disproportionately high among children who are poor, African American, and/or Hispanic.[48] Migrant farmworker children must, therefore, be considered a high-risk population for lead poisoning. Several older studies have documented increased lead exposure in migrant farmworker children, attributed to poor housing and soil contamination.[50,51]

Sources of Lead

Because of their normal oral exploratory behavior, children absorb most lead by ingestion.[49]

- **Lead-based paint** continues to be the principal source of high-dose lead exposure for children. An estimated 57 million housing units in the United States contain lead-based paint. Children are at especially high risk of absorbing lead from paint when housing is poor and deteriorated and paint has chipped, peeled, or cracked; these conditions exist in an estimated 3.8 million US homes with young children.[52] Children may directly absorb lead from paint by ingesting paint chips (pica) or, more commonly, by ingestion of lead-contaminated house dust.

- **Contaminated dust and soil** are pervasive sources of lead exposure.[52] Concentrations of lead in dust and soil range from near zero to many thousands of parts per million (ppm). Lead in dust and soil appears to produce elevations in children's blood lead levels when the concentration exceeds 300 to 500 ppm.

- **Drinking water** is a common source of low-level lead exposure.[52] Although high concentrations of lead in drinking water occurs only in unusual circumstances (such as storage of water in lead-lined tanks), lead in water contributes widely to background exposure. At its source, drinking water is almost always lead-free. Water can, however, become con- taminated as it passes through lead pipes or comes into con- tact with lead solder or brass faucets. Soft water of low pH poses the greatest hazard because it has the greatest capacity to dissolve lead from pipes and solder.

- **Home remedies and folk medicines** can be a source of lead poisoning. Numerous case reports have documented this hazard,[53] and it appears to be especially common among ethnically isolated groups, including migrant children.

- **Imported ceramics and pottery** may contribute to lead absorption. The hazard becomes especially severe when lead-glazed pottery is used to store acidic foods such as fruit juices or salsa.

Effects of Lead Poisoning

Lead is now recognized to produce a wide range of toxicity. These toxic effects extend from acute, clinically obvious poisoning to subclinical effects.[47]

- **Acute poisoning** can be caused by intense exposure to lead, characterized by abdominal colic, constipation, fatigue, anemia, peripheral neuropathy, and alteration of central ner- vous system function.[47] In severe cases, a full-blown acute encephalopathy with coma, convulsions, and papilledema may occur. In milder cases, only headache or personality changes are evident.[47] Children who have recovered from acute lead encephalopathy often are left with permanent neurologic and behavioral sequelae.[52,53]

- **Lower-dose exposures** to lead produce toxic effects, which are typically asymptomatic and become evident only on special testing. These effects are evident principally in the following three organ systems: the developing red blood cells, the kidneys, and the nervous system. Hypochromic microcytic anemia, often associated with iron deficiency, is the classic hematologic manifestation of lead poisoning. High lead levels also can produce basophilic stippling in red blood cells. In the kidneys, acute lead poisoning can produce a full-blown, but reversible, Fanconi syndrome. Chronic, low-dose exposure can produce renal fibrosis and hypertension.

- **Asymptomatic impairment to the nervous system** has been shown by extensive research to be caused by lead at levels too low to produce obvious encephalopathy. Asymptomatic school-aged children with elevated lead levels have been found to have significant decrements in verbal IQ scores.[52] This finding was still strongly evident after adjusting for a wide range of socioeconomic, behavioral, and biologic factors. Long-term follow-up of asymptomatic school-aged children with elevated lead levels has shown that they are at increased risk during adolescence for dyslexia, failure to graduate from high school, and delinquency.[53]

- **Early developmental delays:** Most recently, a series of prospective studies of newborns[49,54] has found associations between early developmental delays and umbilical cord blood lead levels as low as 10 to 20 µg/dL. These findings, which are highly credible, have been accepted by the CDC[49] and by the National Academy of Sciences,[54] and are the basis for the CDC recommendation that the blood lead level of concern in children is 10 µg/dL.[49]

Medical Evaluation

Two fundamental principles must guide assessment of lead exposure in migrant farmworker children.

1. All migrant children 0 to 6 years of age must be considered to be at high risk of lead poisoning. Their high-risk status reflects their poverty and especially their residence in substandard housing that may contain lead paint.

2. Because most pediatric lead poisoning today is asymptomatic, the only reliable means for establishing or excluding a diagnosis of lead poisoning is through determination of the blood lead level. Neither the medical history nor the physical examination can establish or exclude a diagnosis of lead poisoning. Blood for lead analysis may be obtained either by a fingerprick or venipuncture. If a blood lead level greater than or equal to 10 µg/dL is found by a fingerprick, it must be confirmed by venipuncture. The erythrocyte protoporphyrin (EP) test is no longer considered a reliable diagnostic tool for lead poisoning.

Note: All migrant farmworker children 0 to 6 years of age should receive a minimum of two lead tests — one at approximately 1 year of age and the second at age 2. If the blood lead level is greater than or equal to 10 µg/dL in either of these evaluations, if a sibling has elevated blood lead levels, or if the health care professional suspects that a child is exposed to lead, then additional and more frequent blood lead determinations are indicated.

Diagnosis and Plan

A confirmed venous blood lead level in a child of 10 µg/dL or greater establishes a diagnosis of lead poisoning. The management of a child with an elevated blood lead level depends upon the magnitude of the elevation. The following plan is adapted from the 1997 CDC statement,[49] and from guidelines issued by the American Academy of Pediatrics:[55]

- If a child's blood lead level is **between 10 and 25 µg/dL,** medical treatment is not necessary. However, a vigorous search must be made for the source(s) of lead exposure, and the child must be separated from those sources immediately. Sources to be considered include lead paint in all homes and child care settings visited by the child. Soil, dust, drinking water, ceramics, and folk medicines must be considered as well. The child should be followed with frequent blood lead determinations until the clinician is assured that further exposure will not occur. Siblings 0 to 6 years of age and other children living in the same location also need to be evaluated. The parents and guardians need to be carefully educated about the sources of lead that are hazardous to children.

- Children with blood lead levels of **25 to 45 µg/dL** need aggressive environmental intervention, but should not routinely receive chelation therapy because there is no evidence that chelation prevents or reverses subclinical neurotoxicity. If blood lead levels stay elevated despite repeated environmental study and abatement, some children may benefit from (oral) chelation therapy.

- Chelation therapy is indicated in children with blood lead levels **between 45 and 70 µg/dL.** In the absence of clinical symptoms suggesting encephalopathy (eg, obtundation, headache, and persistent vomiting), children may be treated with oral Dimercaptosuccinic Acid (DMSA) at 30 mg/kg/day for 5 days, followed by 20 mg/kg/day for 14 days. To monitor for adverse effects and to permit environmental abatement, children may need to be hospitalized for at least the period of initiation of their therapy. Children should not be discharged from the hospital until their environment has been made lead safe and all lead dust has been removed.

- Children with blood lead levels of **greater than 70 µg/dL** or with clinical symptoms suggesting encephalopathy require immediate inpatient chelation therapy using the most effective parenteral agents. **Lead encephalopathy is a life-threatening emergency.**

- After chelation therapy, a period of re-equilibration of 10 to 14 days should be allowed and then another blood lead level obtained. Repeat courses of oral chelation should be administered as necessary.

The long-term goal of management is to prevent recurrence of lead poisoning in the affected child and also to prevent poisoning in siblings and in playmates. The worst tragedy is to discharge a child home after treatment only to have lead poisoning recur because the child is reexposed.

Pesticide Poisoning

Background

More than 600 chemicals are registered in the United States as pesticides. These include insecticides, herbicides, fungicides, nematocides, and rodenticides. After doubling between the 1960s and 1980s to more than 1 billion pounds per year, pesticide use has since stabilized. An Environmental Protection Agency (EPA) survey estimated that 84% of American households use pesticides — most commonly insecticides. Nearly half of those households with a child younger than 5 years of age has a pesticide stored within reach.

Reasons for Children's Unique Susceptibility to Pesticide Poisoning

- Behaviors related to developmental stages (hand to mouth in toddlers)
- Higher minute ventilation, higher fluid consumption, different diets
- Decreased ability to detoxify some substances
- Rapidly developing neurologic system
- Large body surface area contact with floors, dirt, gardens, etc

---

While specific data on migrant children's exposure to pesticides is very limited, the US EPA has estimated that pesticide exposure causes up to 300,000 acute illnesses and injuries to farmworkers each year. In a recent study in a California agricultural community, pesticides were frequently found in household dust. The highest levels were found in farmworkers' houses and on the hands of toddlers. Children's exposures from different sources (eg, diet, household use, playing, or working in fields) may be cumulative. In recent years, inappropriate and illegal indoor use of agricultural-strength pesticides has been recognized as a serious problem.

Possible Routes of Exposure to Pesticides

- **Dermal.** Many pesticides are readily absorbed through the skin, causing systemic and local irritant effects.
- **Inhalation.** Living near agricultural spraying increases potential for drift exposure. After application, fields and orchards may provide continued airborne exposure for some time.
- **Unintentional Ingestion.** Seventy-five percent of children seen in medical settings for pesticide exposure result from unintentional ingestion.

Diagnosis of Acute Poisoning

Symptoms of acute pesticide poisoning are frequently nonspecific, and laboratory tests often are not diagnostically helpful. Therefore, the history is of particular importance. Children of farmworkers may be exposed to regular consumer products used at home, agricultural products inappropriately used around the house, recent applications in the field, or by playing or working on machinery with pesticide residues. They also may be exposed through contact with working parents who are covered with pesticide residue.

Organophosphate and N-methyl carbamate poisonings are the exception in that they have associated specific symptoms from inhibition of acetylcholinesterase. Remember the mnemonic **DUMBELS**

Diarrhea (abdominal cramps)

Urination (excessive or uncontrolled)

Miosis (pinpoint pupils, though 10% may have mydriasis)

Bradycardia, bronchorrhea, bronchospasm

Excitation/irritability, disorientation

Lacrimation

Salivation

These symptoms of organophosphate and carbamate poisoning are described as "all faucets on," including rhinorrhea, bronchorrhea, and sweating. While adults generally have bradycardia, children with serious poisoning often present with tachycardia and may have seizures. Mild poisoning may produce only nonspecific symptoms such as headache, nausea, vomiting, and dizziness. Examples of organophosphate and N-methyl carbamate pesticides are listed in Table 2-5.

Table 2-5 Examples of Organophosphate (OP) and N-methyl Carbamate Pesticides (C)					
High Toxicity LD50 <50 mg/kg		Moderate Toxicity LD50 50-500 mg/kg		Low Toxicity LD50 >500 mg/kg	
Mevinphos (Phosdrin)	OP	Diazinon	OP	Malathion	OP
Methyl parathion	OP	Chlorpyrifos	OP	Methyl chlorpyrifos	OP
Phorate (Thimet)	OP	(Dursban, Lorsban)		Acephate (Orthene)	OP
Terbufos (Counter, Contraven)	OP	Propoxur (Baygon)	C	Carbaryl (Sevin)	C
Aldicarb (Temik)	C				
Carbofuran (Furadan)	C				

From Morgan D, Reigart JR, Roberts JR, eds. *Recognition and Management of Pesticide Poisonings, 5th ed.* Washington, DC: US Environmental Protection Agency; 1999

The details of treating such poisoning are beyond the scope of this book. Serious poisonings should be managed with guidance from your regional poison control center. The box on the following page provides general guidelines.

**Diagnosis and Treatment of Acute Poisoning
by Organophosphates and N-methyl Carbamates**

1. Obtain a history of exposure.

2. Assess the presence of symptoms of acetylcholine excess (see previous page). Observe closely if asymptomatic or only minor symptoms.

3. If symptomatic, a test dose of atropine supports the diagnosis by *failing* to produce the signs of atropinization (dilation of pupils, dry mouth, flushed skin, increase in heart rate, fever).

4. Draw red blood count and plasma cholinesterase activity with organophosphates but not carbamates. Large variation of individual normal values may require comparison to normal values after recovery. Do not delay treatment while awaiting results.

5. Treat with atropine titrated to control bronchorrhea (drying of secretions and clear lungs) and other symptoms.

6. Pralidoxime (2-Pam) is specific antidote for organophosphates. It is generally not used for carbamates due to serious side effects.

Exposure to paraquat may be confirmed by a simple colorimetric test of urine and may be available from some labs. Plasma paraquat concentrations may be obtained from ICI Americas, Inc., by calling 800/327-8633.

There is no lab confirmation of poisoning for most other pesticides although, for a very few pesticides, blood levels or urine metabolites may be available from specialized labs. Symptoms are generally nonspecific and vary from allergic, respiratory, dermatologic problems, and dermatitis in pyrethrins, to neurobehavioral symptoms, irritant dermatitis, eye damage, and renal and pulmonary disease. Generally, oral ingestions are more likely to be serious, but large amounts of toxicants may be absorbed dermally.

Management

1. **Always try to get the product label!** Do not depend on memory! Relying on memory may result in mistakes because many pesticides have confusingly similar names. Products may change ingredients but retain the same brand name. The EPA-mandated label contains specific information on toxicity, signs, symptoms, treatment, and a manufacturer's toll-free number.

2. **Get help by telephone** for pesticide identification, symptoms, and treatment from

   - Your regional poison control center
   - The National Pesticide Telecommunications Network by calling 800/858-7377 (for health professionals)
   - Your county cooperative extension agent or agricultural commissioner, who may help in identification through their extensive knowledge of local chemical usage

3. **Consult a reference text.** *Recognition and Management of Pesticide Poisonings* is a standard reference that should be available in the emergency department. It includes toxicology, symptoms, and treatment. The chapter "Index to Pesticide Poisonings by Signs and Symptoms," may be helpful with unknown poisoning. An additional reference is *Clinical Management of Poisoning and Drug Overdose.*

4. **If in a hospital emergency department,** do the following:

   - Decontaminate patient and staff by removing clothing, showering, and using protective equipment.
   - Provide immediate cardiopulmonary resuscitation, gastric lavage, and adsorbent as needed.
   - Find out if others are exposed.
   - Significant poisonings should be treated in consultation with a medical toxicologist.
   - When uncertain about the significance of the exposure, observe in hospital for 24 hours.

Preventive Counseling

Exposure assessment and counseling about safe practices should be a part of the health maintenance visit for farmworker children. Stress that following safety precautions will safeguard the entire family's health. Also, work with local farm employers to assist in properly educating families of these hazards.

Encourage Families to Avoid These Unsafe Pesticide Practices

- Do not enter a field that has been posted with a sign indicating pesticide treatment. Treated fields should not be entered by anyone until pesticide dust has settled and plants are dry from spray, unless the worker is wearing protective clothing.

- Do not use water in drainage ditches or any irrigation system for drinking, washing food or clothing, swimming, or fishing.

- Do not put pesticides in unmarked containers or in food or drink jars.

- Never take pesticide containers home for use around the house. They are unsafe.

- Do not burn pesticide bags for fuel; they can give off poisonous fumes.

- Do not use pesticides from work in and around the house.

Encourage Families to Use These Safe Pesticide Practices

- Wash work clothes separately from other laundry.

- Wash work clothes with detergent and hot water before wearing them again.

- Wash hands and arms after putting clothing into washing machine.

- Change clothing and wash with soap and water before picking up or playing with children.

- Store pesticides in an area safe from children.

- Cover children's skin if they are with you at work.

- Keep children and their toys indoors when there is nearby aerial spraying or spraying that may drift near the house.
- Children and teenagers should avoid work that involves spraying or mixing pesticides.

Adapted from INFO Letter: Environmental and Occupational Health Briefs. Vol 9, no 4, 1996. Agrichemicals: the dose makes the poison. Environmental and Health Risk Communication Division. Piscataway, NJ. (See Resources.)

Groundwater Contamination

Background

Half of the country uses groundwater to supply household drinking water. In rural migrant farm camps, this practice may be close to universal. Groundwater wells are prone to contamination from coliform bacteria, nitrates, and pesticides. A camp's water system falls under federal Safe Drinking Water Act standards if piped water is supplied to at least 25 people or 15 service connections for at least 60 days per year. However, compliance is low. In 1991, for instance, the EPA found 191 California migrant camp water systems (of an estimated 300 statewide) in violation either for contamination or failure to monitor.

Physicians and advocates should encourage local public health officials to monitor these wells. Testing for coliforms and nitrates should be accompanied by testing for pesticides. Water from irrigation systems or ditches should not be used for drinking, washing, or laundering.

Nitrate Contamination

Nitrate contamination of rural groundwater in agricultural areas is widespread. Nitrates contaminate well water from agricultural fertilizers, barnyard runoff, and septic systems. A survey of more than 600 wells in Iowa showed 18.3% in excess of 10 ppm (the drinking water standard limit).[56] Excess ingestion of nitrates causes methemoglobinemia. Infants younger than 6 months of age are at greatest risk.

Children with methemoglobinemia have cyanosis with a brownish cast and normal pulse oximetry. The definitive test is the proportion of methemoglobin to hemoglobin. (*See Table 2-6 for a list of the signs and symptoms associated with increasing methemoglobinemia.*)

Table 2-6 Signs and Symptoms Associated With Increasing Methemoglobinemia			
Asymptomatic 3% to 10%	**Mild Toxicity 10% to 30%**	**Moderate Toxicity 30% to 50%**	**Severe Toxicity More Than 50%**
Cyanosis	Headache Fatigue	Headache Weakness Tachypnea Tachycardia Vasodilatation	Stupor Bradycardia Respiratory depression Acidosis Seizures

From American Academy of Pediatrics Committee on Environmental Health. *Handbook of Pediatric Environmental Health.* Elk Grove Village, IL: American Academy of Pediatrics; 1999:166

Recommendation

If a well is unmonitored or not in compliance with drinking water standards, bottled water should be advised, especially for infants younger than 6 months of age. Boiling water tends to increase the concentration of nitrates and is not safe for bottle-fed infants. Inexpensive charcoal water filters are not effective in reducing nitrates.

Child Maltreatment

Background

Working with migrant farmworkers and child maltreatment issues is a difficult and complex task. The pediatrician must have an understanding of multiple child maltreatment considerations (eg, indicators of abuse, injuries consistent with a type of maltreatment, etc), and must appreciate the factors unique to farmworkers (eg, immigration status, language barriers, patterns of health care service utilization). Difficulties may arise due to the family not wanting services, or they may fear seeking, or have difficulty obtaining, services.

It is important to understand that migrant farmworkers and their families may have a poor or small social support network and, thus, may feel isolated. This lack of family and parental support, may put migrant children at increased risk for neglect and/or abuse. Stressors such as being in a new country, lack of understanding of state institutions and regulations, lack of education, and different perceptions about family functioning also can lead to abuse and/or neglect.

When abuse and/or neglect is brought to the attention of health professionals and a child is brought in for services, the parent(s) may not understand the problem (eg, what they determined was appropriate discipline might actually be abuse), and/or they may not have an understanding of the benefits and uses of the health care system in the United States. There also may be reluctance to seek medical services because of perceptions that they cannot afford such health care. Finally, if members of the family do not have clear residency status, there may be concerns about being reported to the Immigration and Naturalization Service.

All 50 states have some type of legal mandate to report "reasonable suspicion" of child maltreatment. Typically, the requirement to report child abuse supersedes issues of patient confidentiality. Child abuse reporting mandates vary by state; it is strongly recommended that pediatricians become familiar with the child abuse reporting mandates for their state.

Assessment

In assessing and managing family problems related to child neglect, it is essential that pediatricians attend to the socioeconomic status of the migrant family. Many problems associated with child neglect mimic the problems of poverty, which is common among migrant farmworker families. Additionally, children may not have access to many health care benefits (eg, consistent dental care, immunizations) that are typical of nonmigrant families or families not in poverty. While the health status of these children is no less important, parents should not be blamed for problems that are beyond their resources. Medical neglect may be a consequence of the migrant lifestyle and the lack of available health care services.

As physicians working with migrant farmworkers, it is very important to assess the following areas:

- **Legal Factors.** The migrant farmworker and his or her family may not be aware of the laws surrounding mandated child abuse reporting. As physicians, it is very important to inform the patient of such laws and what the physician is obligated to do under such circumstances.

- **Cultural Factors.** There are many cultural factors that should be taken into consideration when working with migrant farmworkers. Most importantly, physicians should assess for level of acculturation. This can be done by assessing the following:

  - Generation status of the child(ren) and parents
  - Family members' educational level and country of education
  - Language preference with regard to reading, writing, and speaking; English proficiency
  - Religious beliefs and practices
  - Beliefs about relevant issues such as health care, family structure, discipline practices, parenting roles, the child's role in the family, and gender roles for different family members

- **Poverty.** Usually, migrant farmworkers live in impoverished and high-risk neighborhoods. There may be a lack of food, heat, electricity, and running water. If both parents work, there may be a lack of child care for the children. The family also may be sharing a house or apartment with several other extended family members and/or nonrelated families. Resources for discipline, such as "time out" locations, must be understood. The child's sleeping arrangements should be noted as well.

- **Spiritual/Religious Beliefs.** Such beliefs can be helpful or harmful in terms of seeking and accepting health care services. As an example, some patients may be inclined to seek traditional healing practices such as consulting with family or highly regarded community members, or wanting to use herbs as healing remedies. They also may want to leave the situation in "God's hands" and thus not seek services. These practices are not inherently wrong, but are important areas of assessment.

Intervention

Services offered should be as culturally relevant as possible, community-based, and available in the language the family speaks. The scheduling of services is important to consider because many families cannot afford to leave work for appointments during the day or anytime during the work week. Parenting workshops may be held in Spanish at a local meeting place that is utilized by the migrant farmworkers (eg, a church in the community or a Head Start provider). Physicians must educate the patient on the services offered and why they are relevant. Other issues, such as needing to provide vouchers for transportation and child care services for the other children while the parent attends classes, also are important to address.

Injuries

Background

Injuries are the most common cause of death during childhood beyond the first few months of life and represent one of the most important causes of preventable pediatric morbidity and mortality. Children of farmworkers are at risk for injuries from the usual hazards facing all children, as well as the special hazards inherent in agricultural work. Among adolescent workers, agriculture is one of the most dangerous occupations.[57] Reduction in morbidity and mortality from injuries can be accomplished not only through primary prevention of the injury, but also through secondary and tertiary prevention. This includes appropriate emergency medical services for children, a special issue in rural areas. These services should include regionalized trauma care for children with multiple injuries, burns, and head trauma, and specialized pediatric rehabilitation services that attempt to return the injured child to his or her prior level of functioning. This broadened scope of prevention is more properly described by the term *injury control.*

Magnitude of the Problem

Accurate data on farm injuries are difficult to obtain. A number of studies have found that death certificate data do not completely capture all injuries.[58,59] Data on injuries to farmworker children are currently unavailable. No surveillance studies of injuries in this population have been conducted. Death certificate data or data from hospital discharge databases do not distinguish farmworkers or their children from the general population. A major tenet of public health is that to prevent morbidity or mortality, a public health problem must be diagnosed and understood. Our lack of data on injuries to farmworker children thus represents a major problem. Available data indicate that approximately 100 children per year die on farms in the United States due to agriculture-related injuries, and an additional 27,000 children are injured seriously enough to require emergency department treatment.[60]

Injuries that occur on farms tend to be more severe than those occurring in other occupations. Among workers 13 years of age or younger in Washington state, farmwork accounted for 50% of all severe injury claims and for 48% of all disabling injury claims, compared with 5% and 7%, respectively, among food service workers.[61]

Finally, all of the data on injuries focus on acute trauma; data on the incidence of chronic problems, such as back pain from stooping and lifting, are unavailable. Yet, musculoskeletal complaints rank high in surveys of health problems of farmworkers.[62]

Types of Injuries

Most of the severe and fatal injuries on the farm are related to **machinery.**[58,63-65] This appears to be true for children and adolescents as well as adults. In most studies, tractors are responsible for the most injuries (especially severe and fatal injuries) involving machinery.[58,66,67] This is due to a combination of rollovers, as well as injuries from the power-take-off device. Rollover incidents accounted for 46% of all farm tractor-related fatalities in Minnesota, 76% in Georgia,[68] and 82% in Kentucky.[66]

Power-take-off devices, which are common pieces of farm machinery, have the potential to produce severe injuries such as avulsions and amputations; yet many farmers remove the protective cover on these devices to facilitate use and repair.

Children are at particular risk for **animal**-related injuries on farms, and animals are one of the most common sources of injuries to female children on farms.[64,69] Overall, animals account for 17% of agriculture-related injuries.[62] These injuries usually involve being stepped on or kicked by horses or livestock.

Farms require the use of many **chemicals** that are potentially dangerous. The hazards of organophosphate pesticides are well known. *(See Environmental Concerns section.)* One chemical that is used particularly on dairy farms is caustic alkali. Ingestion of this chemical usually occurs in young children and can result in severe injury.[70] Most commonly, the chemical has been taken out if its original container and placed in another smaller container for daily use, resulting in easier access and ingestion by small children.

Falls are a frequent cause of injuries on the farm, most commonly from barns and haymows. Interestingly, adults who care for preschoolers on farms have a risk of fall injury two and a half times greater than those who do not care for children.[71]

Violence is one area of injury in farmworker children that has not received adequate attention. The actual incidence of injuries from violence in this population is unknown because of inadequate data collection. However, one survey of seasonal and migrant farmworker families with 8- to 11-year-old children found that exposure to violence was common.[72] Forty-six percent of these children had been witnesses to violence, including 20% being witnesses to a shooting and 11% being witnesses to a murder. One in five children of this age group were victims of violence, with many of the victims also being witnesses. As expected, children who witness violence are more likely than other children to have behavioral problems. Nearly one third of the children between 8 and 11 years of age who were exposed to violence carried weapons.

The Screening History: Risk Factors for Injuries

In taking a history, an assessment of risk is required. Risks for injuries are best considered in an epidemiological framework of host, agent, and environment. The environment also can be further categorized as the physical environment and the sociocultural environment.

- **Host.** For many years, the common response to an accident resulting in injury has been to blame it on some incorrect behavior or activity of the victim. This generally has been unproductive in devising intervention strategies and may not be a particularly fruitful area for clinicians. In addition, we know little about actual risk behavior in those who are injured compared with those who are uninjured, and almost nothing about such behavior in children of farmworkers. One study found that immigrant and native Hispanic high school students had higher rates of self-reported alcohol use, drunk driving, and fighting than did native non-Hispanic whites.[73] These behaviors potentially could affect the risk of non–farm-related injuries, but their affect on risk of agriculturally related injuries is unknown.

> Males have higher rates of farm-related injuries compared with females at all ages.[69] This is almost certainly due to exposure; ie, males are more likely to be working on farms and around equipment. Among adolescents, the majority of injuries are due to work.[57] Unfortunately, accurate exposure data for children and adolescents are lacking.

- **Agent.** Agents of injury are ubiquitous on farms. Farm vehicles, tractors, electrical tools, and sharp tools are present on nearly every farm.[74] Power hand tools are used on most farms, as are various chemicals such as pesticides, herbicides, caustics, and other poisons. Unfortunately, many of the safeguards for these pieces of equipment are not used, either because they have been purposely removed, have broken and not been repaired, or did not exist in the first place.[63,74] Machinery is often not replaced until it is very old and beyond repair. Rollover protection structures (ROPS) are the best means of preventing death from tractors, decreasing deaths by approximately 43%.[68] Although virtually all new tractors sold in the United States since 1985 have been equipped with ROPS, an eight-state survey of tractors found that 65% of tractors had no rollover protection. A recent survey found that 30% of boys on farms are driving tractors by age 7 to 9, and 95% are riding on them.[69]

- **Physical Environment.** Farming is unique in that children are living in an environment in which large machinery is used. This is true of no other industry; children do not live on a factory floor, for example. This exposure to hazards creates risks to children of all ages, including very young children under the age of 5 for whom child care commonly does not exist. The environment also plays a role in the outcome of injury once it occurs. Trauma care in rural areas is less well-developed than in urban areas, arrival times of paramedics are longer, and definitive care often requires transfer to an urban center. This decreased access to care can result in higher morbidity and mortality.[75,76] Definitive pediatric trauma care is particularly rare in rural areas.

> A survey of injuries in New York state found that the majority of agricultural injuries to adolescents occurred on dairy farms (39%), crop-producing farms (37%), and in auxiliary agricultural services (17%).[57]

- **Sociocultural Environment.** One of the major reasons for the continued toll of injuries in agriculture is that Occupational Safety and Health Administration (OSHA) regulations are not enforced on farms with fewer than 11 employees, which account for the majority of farms in the United States, and certainly the majority of those with migrant farmworkers. Thus, compliance with requirements such as ROPS on tractors will be poor on many such farms where economics dictate extending the life of machinery and tools as long as possible. In addition, there are no legal injury-reporting requirements for farms with fewer than 11 employees, resulting in little data being available. Clinicians should consider reporting severe injuries to the state occupational safety and health office.

Child labor laws for agriculture are quite different from those for other industries (a difference dating back to 1932). The federal legal age to work on nonfamily farms is 12 years and minors younger than 12 may be employed in nonhazardous work on small farms with the consent of their parents.[69] In contrast, the legal age limit for other industries is 16 years, and for hazardous work, 18 years. It is not known how many children of migrant farmworkers are formally employed. Many work alongside older family members, contributing to the adult wage earner's harvest without individually receiving compensation.

Injury Control Strategies

Control of injuries to children of farmworkers must rest on a combination of education; legislation; product modification; environmental modification; and improvements in access to, and quality of, medical care. While the clinician is most logically involved with care and rehabilitation of the injured child, involvement in prevention also is appropriate, if not necessary. The National Committee for Childhood Agricultural Injury Prevention has developed a list of recommendations for action *(see box on opposite page)*, and these should be the basis of a national agenda for a reduction of morbidity and mortality from these injuries. The National Children's Center for Rural and Agricultural Health and Safety also has developed a set of guidelines for parents, employers, and health professionals, called the "North American Guidelines for Children's Agricultural Tasks — Guidelines." The guidelines help adults match a child's physical, mental, and emotional abilities with the requirements of agricultural jobs. *(See Resources.)*

Recommendations of the National Committee for Childhood Agricultural Injury Prevention

1. Establish and maintain a national system for childhood agricultural injury prevention.

2. Ensure that childhood agricultural injury prevention programs are supported with sufficient funding and cooperation from the public and private sectors.

3. Establish guidelines for children's and adolescents' work in the industry of agriculture.

4. Ensure that the public is aware of general childhood agricultural safety and health issues.

5. Establish and maintain a comprehensive national database of fatal and nonfatal childhood agricultural injuries.

6. Conduct research on costs, risk factors, and consequences associated with children and adolescents who participate in agricultural work.

7. Use systematic evaluations to ensure that educational materials and methods targeted toward childhood agricultural safety and health have demonstrated positive results.

8. Ensure that farm and ranch owner/operators, farmworkers, parents, and caregivers understand relevant agricultural safety and health issues that pertain to children and adolescents.

9. Ensure that rural safety and health professionals understand the issues relevant to children and adolescents exposed to agricultural hazards.

10. Influence adult behaviors that affect protection of children and adolescents through the use of incentives and adoption of voluntary guidelines.

11. Provide a protective and supportive environment for children exposed as bystanders to agricultural hazards.

12. Establish uniform standards that address the protection of children and adolescents from agricultural occupational hazards.

13. Increase adherence to child labor laws through active and funded enforcement, including the use of penalties.

National Committee for Childhood Agricultural Injury Prevention. Children and agriculture: opportunities for safety and health. Marshfield, WI: Marshfield Clinic; 1996.

The clinician should specifically intervene through **education and advocacy** to decrease the risk of injury to migrant farmworker children.

- Parents should be advised not to bring children to the fields and not to allow them around dangerous machinery and chemicals. This must be accompanied by advocacy to make child care accessible and available for these children as a feasible alternative.

- For school-aged children, the clinician should counsel parents about the negative impact of working, especially more than 20 hours per week, on the child's education and success in school. Education remains the great equalizer in the United States; sacrificing the child's education for the immediate financial rewards of the child's work may condemn the youngster to a life of unskilled labor.

- Children who are working in the fields should be assessed as to their risks and appropriate interventions offered. Adolescents exposed to farm machinery should take locally available extension service courses on farm machinery safety, safe lifting techniques, and safe use of agriculture chemicals.

The clinician should be involved in establishing protocols for the proper care of injured children and adolescents. This means equipping the office for handling emergencies, establishing office protocols for the management of seriously injured children, ensuring that the local emergency medical professionals have the proper equipment and training to care for injured children, and ensuring that relationships are established with regional Level I trauma centers for care and rehabilitation of seriously injured children.

Finally, child health care professionals should consider avenues for advocacy to improve the health and welfare of migrant farmworkers and their children. This may take the form of arranging for free child care or of working at the state level on child labor regulations. Pediatricians long have been at the forefront of advocacy to prevent child injury. Prevention of farm injuries to children and adolescents can only be accomplished by pediatricians working in their communities as well as in their offices.

Infectious Diseases

Background

Living and working in substandard conditions puts migrant children at greater risk for developing communicable diseases. Among this population, the death rate for tuberculosis and other communicable diseases is estimated to be 20 to 25 times higher than the national average.[77] Children of migrant farmworkers may harbor infectious diseases that US health care workers may be inexperienced in diagnosing and treating. These include conditions such as malaria, amebiasis, and other parasitic diseases; congenital syphilis, for which foreign-born children are not necessarily screened at birth; and leprosy and tuberculosis. While the *2000 Red Book* is the resource for presentation and management of these diseases, a brief description of each, as it is pertinent in the case of migrant farmworker children, is presented in this chapter.

Tuberculosis

A high incidence of TB among migrant farmworkers has been well documented. Lack of access to health care, as well as poverty, crowded living conditions, and frequent relocation are major components in the complex circumstances that make the prevention and control of TB among this disadvantaged group more difficult. Epidemiologic studies have suggested that TB among farmworkers is an occupational problem, not an imported one.[78]

Rates of tuberculin skin test positivity among migrant farmworkers have ranged from 11% to 44%, with rates as high as 76% for Haitians and 64% for US-born blacks.[78-81] The rate of TB among the children of these migrant workers is not known, but is expected to be high because most children are infected by an infectious adult in the immediate household.

Clinical Manifestation

There are three basic definitions of TB in children.

1. **Exposure.** Exposure implies that the child has had significant contact with an adolescent or adult with contagious pulmonary TB. The most frequent setting for exposure is the household. In this stage, the tuberculin skin test is negative, the chest radiograph is normal, and there are no signs or symptoms. It is not possible to determine if the child is truly infected because it may take up to 3 months after the exposure for the skin test to become positive.

2. **Infection.** The hallmark of TB infection is a reactive Mantoux tuberculin skin test, without signs or symptoms of tuberculosis, and a chest radiograph that is either normal or reveals a calcification.

3. **Disease.** Tuberculosis disease is said to be present when signs or symptoms or radiographic abnormalities caused by *M. tuberculosis* become manifest.

Diagnosis

The Mantoux tuberculin skin test is the only technique acceptable in the evaluation of children. Multiple puncture devices are no longer used because of their inaccuracy. The CDC and the American Academy of Pediatrics have recommended stratification of the size of the induration to be considered positive, depending on the risk factors for that child. *(See the 2000 Red Book.)* For children at the highest risk of infection, a reaction of greater than 5 mm in diameter is classified as positive. For other high-risk groups, a reaction of greater than 10 mm is a positive result. Virtually all children of migrant workers are in one of these two categories.

If the skin test is not adequately explained, some migrants may think it is a vaccination against TB. Pediatric health care professionals need to explain that the skin test is only a *test* to see if TB is present.

In their country of origin, many farmworkers have received a *Bacillus Calmette-Guerin* (BCG) vaccination, which may cause increased reactivity to a subsequent tuberculin skin test, but the association is weaker than many clinicians suspect. In the absence of a clear history, a small scar on the upper arm probably means the child received a BCG vaccination. Studies have shown that fewer than 50% of infants given BCG vaccine at birth have a reactive tuberculin skin test at 6 to 12 months of age, and that virtually all vaccinated infants have nonreactive tests by 5 years of age.[82] Among older children or adults who receive a BCG vaccine, a higher percentage develop a reactive skin test. By 10 to 15 years post-vaccination, most have lost tuberculin skin test reactivity. Studies in migrant workers have confirmed that BCG vaccination may have no influence on PPD reactions.[78] For these reasons, most experts agree that, in general, the previous administration of BCG should not influence the application or interpretation of the tuberculosis skin test.

Management

Because migrant farmworkers are considered to be at increased risk, the Academy recommends skin testing for this group at the time of immigration, and every 2 to 3 years thereafter.[83] They also should be immediately tested if they have radiographic or clinical findings suggestive of tuberculosis, or if they have contacted persons with confirmed or suspected infectious tuberculosis ("contact investigation"). Annual testing is recommended for children infected with HIV or those living in a household with persons infected with HIV.

Refer to the *2000 Red Book* for information related to exposure, treatment, and follow-up of tuberculosis.

Intestinal Parasitic Infestation

Intestinal parasite infestation is considered a major problem among migrant farmworkers who work and live in substandard hygienic conditions. Factors that allow the spread of these infections include exposure to drinking water that is contaminated with these organisms, inadequate toilet facilities, and insufficient washing water to prevent or reduce fecal-oral transmission. In addition, most of these parasitic agents are able to survive in the field (outside the human host) anywhere from 3 weeks to 3 months or more. Prevalence rates for parasites among farmworker populations range from 20% to 86%. The parasite prevalence rate, even among US-born migrant farmworkers, is much higher than that of the general population (28% versus 1% to 3%, respectively).[84] Children are particularly susceptible to parasitic infestation and may serve as sources of reinfection within the family.

Clinical Manifestation

Symptoms of intestinal parasitic infestation are often minimal or vague, but may be more severe with heavier infections. Symptoms that may occur with common parasitic infestations include abdominal discomfort, anorexia, nausea, diarrhea, edema, weight loss, failure to thrive, and malabsorption. Bowel obstruction and death have occurred as a result of severe parasitic infestation. Anal pruritus is common with pinworm (*Enterobius vermicularis*) infestation. Infections with parasites that have pulmonary migration may present with pneumonitis. Hematologic abnormalities that may be seen with parasitic infections include anemia and eosinophilia.

Reserve screening for parasite by stool collection for children who have signs of infection or who are known contacts of infected cases.

Refer to the *2000 Red Book* for specific diagnoses and treatment plans.

Tissue Protozoan Infections (Trypanosomiasis [Chagas' Disease])

American trypanosomiasis (Chagas' disease) is a zoonosis caused by the protozoan parasite *Trypanosoma cruzi*. This disease is endemic in almost all Latin American countries, including Mexico and the Central American nations, where the majority of the migrant farmworkers were born. The prevalence of infection among Central American immigrants is estimated to be around 5%.[85] A small survey done among foreign-born migrant farmworkers and their family members in North Carolina revealed a seroprevalence of 2%.

The incubation period for the acute disease is 1 to 2 weeks after the bite from a triatoma insect (reduviid or "kissing bug") infected with the insect's feces. The chronic manifestations of this disease do not appear for years to decades.

Clinical Manifestation

Acute Chagas' disease is usually a mild illness, but children are more likely than adults to develop symptoms. In some patients, the site of inoculation develops a red nodule (chagoma), with induration and hypopigmentation of the surrounding skin. This may be accompanied by fever, malaise, and edema of the eyelids (Romaña's sign), face, and lower extremities, as well as generalized lymphadenopathy and hepatosplenomegaly. Acute myocarditis and meningoencephalitis may develop in a small number of patients. The acute illness spontaneously resolves after 4 to 6 weeks in most patients.

Chronic Chagas' disease, characterized by cardiomyopathy, heart failure, megaesophagus, and/or megacolon, develops in 10% to 30% of infected persons many years to decades after the acute infection.

Refer to the *2000 Red Book* for laboratory diagnosis and treatment.

Leishmaniasis

Leishmaniasis is a zoonosis caused by different species of the intracellular parasite *Leishmania,* which is transmitted by the bite of the sand fly. This parasite is endemic in areas extending from Mexico to northern Argentina, as well as in the Middle East, Asia, and Africa. The incubation period ranges from several days to months.

Clinical Manifestation

Leishmania may cause three different clinical syndromes.

1. *Cutaneous leishmaniasis* is characterized by an erythematous macule or nodule at the site of the inoculation, sometimes accompanied by satellite lesions and regional adenopathy. The lesion typically develops into a shallow ulcer with

raised borders, taking several weeks to months to resolve spontaneously.

2. *Mucosal leishmaniasis* results from the spread of the parasite to the oral and nasal mucous membranes, which can lead to granulomatous ulceration and perforation of facial structures.

3. *Viceral leishmaniasis* (kala-azar) is seen almost exclusively in the Old World and is characterized by fever, hepatosplenomegaly, lymphadenopathy, pancytopenia, and secondary infections.

Refer to the *2000 Red Book* for laboratory tests and treatment.

Malaria

Malaria remains endemic in many rural areas through southern Mexico, Haiti, and Central America. Several outbreaks of malaria in the United States have occurred among farmworkers, and some have involved the possibility of secondary transmission within local farmworkers' communities.[86,87]

Clinical Manifestation

Plasmodium infection is characterized by high fever and chills, which may be accompanied by headache, nausea, abdominal or back pain, and arthralgia. Hepatosplenomegaly is frequently seen in chronic infections, and anemia and jaundice may be present as a result of hemolysis. Cerebral malaria, renal failure, and vascular collapse are potentially fatal complications of infection due to *P. falciparum*. Though rare, congenital malaria may occur.

Refer to the *2000 Red Book* for laboratory diagnosis and treatment.

Human Immunodeficiency Virus Infection

Infection due to human immunodeficiency virus (HIV) in children may cause a broad spectrum of disease, with acquired immunodeficiency syndrome (AIDS) representing the most severe end of the clinical spectrum. Human immunodeficiency virus can be transmitted by sexual contact, percutaneous exposure to contaminated body fluids, vertical transmission from mother to infant before or around the time of birth, and through breastfeeding. Mother-to-infant transmission accounts for more than 90% of the infected children in the United States. The incubation period for perinatally acquired HIV is shorter than that for infection acquired later in life, and the median age of onset of symptoms is currently estimated to be 3 years, although a significant number of infected infants die before 18 months of age.

The National Commission to Prevent Infant Mortality has estimated that migrant and seasonal farmworkers are contracting HIV at 10 times the rate of the general population, and that many lack access to the prevention, treatment, and educational services that could minimize their risk.[88] Although estimates of the prevalence of HIV infection in this group are limited, small screening programs among migrant farmworkers in Florida and North Carolina have revealed a seroprevalance of 2.6% to 5%.[89,90] In addition to the risk factors of the general population, the self-injection of vitamins and antibiotics and needle sharing seem to be widespread among migrant workers, further increasing the risk for HIV transmission.[91]

Clinical manifestation, laboratory diagnosis, and treatment plans are found in the *2000 Red Book* and the October 1998 issue of *Pediatrics.*

Congenital Syphilis

As with many other sexually transmitted diseases, the prevalence of syphilis is higher among migrant farmworkers than that of the general population. A serologic survey among migrant farmworkers done in Florida in 1992 revealed a seroprevalence of 8%.[92] Poor accessibility to prenatal care for this population favors an increase in the rate of congenital syphilis. Additionally, some affected children might have escaped diagnosis, as prenatal screening of syphilis is not mandatory in many of their countries of origin.

See the *2000 Red Book* for laboratory testing, evaluation, and treatment.

Leprosy (Hansen's Disease)

Leprosy is a chronic bacterial disease of the skin, peripheral nerves, and the mucosa of the upper respiratory tract due to *Mycobacterium leprae*. The major mode of transmission is by close contact with an untreated lepromatous patient, probably through nasal secretions. Children are particularly susceptible to this infection. The overcrowded housing conditions of the migrant community may favor the spread of the disease, as household and prolonged close contact are important for its transmission. In the United States, 90% of reported cases are imported from endemic areas, particularly Southeast Asia, Mexico, Brazil, and Colombia.[93] It is estimated that only 25% of the imported cases are patients known to have had leprosy at the time of immigration, so the majority of cases are diagnosed in this country. The incubation period for the disease ranges from 1 to many years (average 3 to 5 years).

See the *2000 Red Book* for Clinical Manifestation, diagnostic tests, and treatment plans.

References

1. American Academy of Pediatrics Ad Hoc Task Force on Definition of the Medical Home. The medical home. *Pediatrics*. 1992;90:774
2. National Commission on Migrant Education. *Invisible Children: A Portrait of Migrant Education in the United States*. Washington, DC: National Commission on Migrant Education; 1992
3. National Association of State Directors of Migrant Education. *Giving Migrant Students an Opportunity to Learn*. Sunnyside, Calif: National Association of Migrant Educators; 1994
4. National Preschool Coordination Project. *Visions: The Newsletter of the National Preschool Coordination Project* 1990-1993; 1(1-5), 2(15). San Diego, Calif: National Preschool Coordination Project

5. National Preschool Coordination Project. *Developmentally and Culturally Appropriate Practices: Burning Issues Series.* Sacramento, Calif: California State Department of Education; 1991

6. US Department of Education. *Strong Families, Strong Schools: A Research Base for Family Involvement in Learning From the US Department of Education.* Washington, DC: US Department of Education; 1994

7. Wiecha JM, Gann P. Does maternal prenatal care use predict infant immunization delay? *Fam Med.* 1994;26:172-178

8. Martin PL. *Migrant Farmworkers and their Children.* Charleston, WVa: Clearinghouse on Rural Education and Small Schools (ED 376 997). 1994

9. Appalachia Educational Laboratory, 1994. *Findings From the National Agricultural Workers Survey (NAWS) 1989: A Demographic and Employment Profile of Perishable Crop Farmworkers.* Washington, DC: US Department of Labor; 1991. Office of Program Economics, Research Report 2

10. Bechtel GA, Shepherd M, Rogers PW. Family, culture and health practices among migrant farm workers. *Community Health Nurs.* 1995;12:15-22

11. Fitzpatrick SB, Fuji C, Schragg GP. Do health care needs of indigent Mexican-American, Black and white adolescents differ? *Adolesc Health Care.* 1990;11:128-132

12. American Medical Association. *Guidelines for Adolescent Preventive Services (GAPS).* Chicago, Ill: American Medical Association, 1994

13. Siantz ML. The Mexican-American migrant farmworker family: Mental-Health Issues. *Nurs Clin North Am.* 1994;29:65-72

14. Reynoso TC, Felice ME, Shragg GP. Does American acculturation affect outcome of Mexican-American teenage pregnancy? *J Adolesc Health.* 1993;14:257-261

15. Nidorf, JF, Morgan MC. Cross cultural issues in adolescent medicine. *Prim Care.* 1987;14:69-82

16. Felice ME, Jenkins R. Cross-Cultural Youth. In: McAnarney ER, Kreipe RE, Orr DP, Comerci GD. *Textbook of Adolescent Medicine*. Philadelphia, Pa: WB Saunders; 1992: pp 214-217

17. Dever A. Migrant health status profile of a population with complex health problems. *Tex J Rural Health*. 1992;6-27

18. Acs G, Lodolini G, Kaminsky S, Cisneros G. Effect of nursing caries on body weight in a pediatric population. *Pediatr Dent*. 1992;14:302-305

19. Duncan B, Ey J, Holberg CJ, Wright AL, Martinez FD, Taussig LM. Exclusive breast-feeding for at least four months protects against otitis media. *Pediatrics*. 1993;91:867-872

20. Narayanan I, Singh S, Mathur R, Jain BK. Ear infection and infant feeding practices. *Indian J Pediatr*. 1989;56:399-402

21. Call R, Entwistle B, Swanson T. Dental caries in permanent teeth in children of migrant farm workers. *Am J Pediatr Health*. 1987;77:1002-1003

22. Koday M, Rosenstein D, Lopez G. Dental decay rates among children of migrant workers in Yakima, Washington. *Public Health Rep*. 1990;105:530-533

23. Ragno J, Castaldi CR. Dental health in a group of migrant children in Connecticut. *J Conn State Dent Assoc*. 1982;56:15-21

24. Avery KT. Department of Community Dentistry, University of Florida College of Dentistry, Gainesville, Florida. *Community Dent Oral Epidemiol*. 1976;4:19-21

25. Bachand RG, Gangarosa LP, Bragassa C. A study of dental needs: DMF, def, and tooth eruption in migrant Negro children. *ASDC J Dent Child*. 1971;28:399-403

26. Entwistle BA, Swanson TM. Dental needs and perceptions of adult Hispanic migrant farmworkers in Colorado. *J Dent Hyg*. 1989;63:286-292

27. American Academy of Pediatrics Committee on Nutrition. *Pediatric Nutrition Handbook*, 4th ed. Elk Grove Village, Ill. American Academy of Pediatrics, 1998:525

28. De Bruyn H, Arends J. Fluoride varnishes—a review. *J Bio Buccale.* 1987;15:71-82

29. Anderson MH, Bales DJ, Omnell KA. Modern management of dental caries: the cutting edge is not the dental bur. *J Am Dent Assoc.* 1993;124:36-44

30. Looker AC, Loria CM, Carroll MD, McDowell MA, Johnson CL. Calcium intakes of Mexican Americans, Cubans, Puerto Ricans, non-Hispanic whites, and non-Hispanic blacks in the United States. *J Am Diet Assoc.* 1993;93:1274-1279

31. Guendelman S, Abrams B. Dietary intake among Mexican-American women: generational differences and a comparison with white non-Hispanic women. *Am J Public Health.* 1995;85:20-25

32. Winkleby MA. Hispanic/white differences in dietary fat intake among low education adults and children. *Prev Med.* 1994;23:465-473

33. Young SA, Kaufman M. Promoting breastfeeding at a migrant health center. *Am J Public Health.* 1988;78:523-525

34. Lipsky S, Stephenson PA, Koepsell TD, Gloyd SS, Lopez JL, Bain CE. Breastfeeding and weaning practices in rural Mexico. *Nut Health.*1994;9:255-263

35. Perez-Escamilla R, Roman Perez R, Mejia LA, Deucy KG. Infant feeding practices among low-income Mexican urban women: a four month follow-up. *Arch Latinoam Nutr.* 1992;42:259-267

36. Olvera-Ezzell N, Power TG, Cousins JH, Giverra AM, Trujillo M. The development of health knowledge in low-income Mexican-American children. *Child Dev.* 1994;65:416-427

37. Wolf AM, Gortmaker SL, Cheung L, Gray HM, Herzog DB, Colditz GA. Activity, inactivity, and obesity: racial, ethnic, and age difference among school girls. *Am J Public Health.* 1993;83:1625-1627

38. Watkins El, Larson K, Harlan C, Young S. A model program for providing health services for migrant farmworker mothers and children. *Public Health Rep.* 1990;105:567-575

39. Malina RM. Ethnic variation in the prevalence of obesity in North American children and youth. *Crit Rev Food Sci Nutr.* 1993;33:389-396

40. Must A, Gortmaker SL, Dietz WH. Risk factors for obesity in young adults: Hispanics, African Americans and whites in the transition years, age 16-28 years. *Biomed Pharmacother.* 1994;48:143-156

41. Resnicow K, Futlerman R, Vaughan RD. Body mass index as a predictor of systolic blood pressure in a multiracial sample of US schoolchildren. *Ethn Dis.* 1993;3:351-361

42. Allen LH, Backstrand JR, Stanek EJ III, et al. The interactive effects of dietary quality on the growth and attained size of young Mexican children. *Am J Clin Nutr.* 1992;56:353-364

43. Weissman AM. Preventive health care and screening of Latin American immigrants in the United States. *J Am Board Fam Pract.* 1994;7;310-323

44. Sargent JD, Stokel TA, Dalten MA, Freeman JL, Brown MJ. Iron deficiency in Massachusetts communities: socioeconomic and demographic risk factors among children. *Am J Public Health.* 1996;86:544-550

45. Cousins JH, Rubovits DS, Dunn JK, Reeves RS, Ramirez AG, Foreyt JP. Family versus individually oriented intervention for weight loss in Mexican American women. *Public Health Rep.* 1992;107:549-555

46. Balcazar H, Trier CM, Cobas JA. What predicts breast-feeding intention in Mexican-American and non-Hispanic white women? Evidence from a national survey. *Birth.* 1995;22:74-80

47. Landrigan PJ, Todd AC. Lead poisoning. Review. *West J Med.* 1994;161:153-159

48. Centers for Disease Control and Prevention. Update: Blood lead levels—United States, 1991-1994. *MMWR.* 1997;46:141-146

49. Centers for Disease Control and Prevention. *Screening Young Children for Lead Poisoning: Guidance for State and Local Health Officials.* Atlanta, Ga: Centers for Disease Control and Prevention; 1997

50. Perrin JM, Merken MJ. Blood lead level in a rural population: relative elevations among migrant farmworker children. *Pediatrics*. 1979;64:540-542

51. Osband ME, Tubin JR. Lead paint exposure in migrant labor camps. *Pediatrics*. 1972;49:604-606

52. Mushak P, Crocetti AF. Determination of numbers of lead-exposed American children as a function of lead source: integrated summary of a report to the US Congress on childhood lead poisoning. Review. *Environ Res*. 1989;50:210-229

53. Centers for Disease Control and Prevention. Lead poisoning from lead tetroxide used as a folk remedy. Colorado. *MMWR*. 1982;30:647-648

54. National Research Council. *Measuring Lead Exposure in Infants, Children, and Other Sensitive Populations*. Washington, DC: *National Academy Press;* 1993

55. American Academy of Pediatrics Committee on Environmental Health. Screening for elevated blood lead levels. *Pediatrics*. 1998;101:1072-1078

56. Kross BC, Hallberg GR, Bruner DR, Cherryholmes K. The nitrate contamination of private well water in Iowa. *Am J Public Health*. 1993;83:270-272

57. Belville R, Pollack SH, Godbold JH, Landrigan PJ. Occupational injuries among working adolescents in New York State. *JAMA*. 1993;269:2754-2759

58. Brison R, Pickett W. Fatal farm injuries in Ontario, 1984 through 1992. *Can J Public Health*. 1995;86:246-248

59. Hayden G, Gerberich S, Maldonado G. Fatal farm injuries: a five-year study utilizing a unique surveillance approach to investigate the concordance of reporting between two data sources. *J Occup Environ Med*. 1995;37:571-577

60. Rivara F. Fatal and non-fatal farm injuries to children and adolescents in the United States, 1990-3. *Inj Prev*. 1997:3:190-194

61. Heyer NJ, Franklin G, Rivara FP, Parker P, Haug JA. Occupational injuries among minors doing farm work in Washington state: 1986 to 1989. *Am J Public Health*. 1992;82:557-560

62. Mobed K, Gold E, Schenker M. Occupational health problems among migrant and seasonal farm workers. *West J Med.* 1992;157:367-373

63. Pickett W, Brison R, Neizgoda H, Chipman ML. Nonfatal farm injuries in Ontario: a population-based survey. *Accid Anal Prev.* 1995;27:425-433

64. Young S. Agriculture-related injuries in the park land region of Manitoba. *Canadian Family Physician.* 1995;41:1190-1197

65. Zhou C, Roseman J. Agricultural injuries among a population-based sample of farm operators in Alabama. *Am J Ind Med.* 1994;25:385-402

66. Farm-tractor-related fatalities—Kentucky, 1994. *MMWR Morb Mortal Wkly Rep.* 1995;44:481-484

67. Vanneuville G, Corger H, Tanguy A, Dalens T, Scheye T, Flaucaud D. Severe farm machinery injuries to children—a report on 15 cases. *Eur J Pediatri Surg.* 1992;2:29-31

68. Public health focus: effectiveness of rollover protective structures for preventing injuries associated with agricultural tractors. *MMWR Morb Mortal Wkly Rep.*1993;42:57-59

69. Wilk V. Health hazards to children in agriculture. *Am J Ind Med.* 1993;24:283-290

70. Neidich, G. Ingestion of caustic alkali farm products. *J Pediatr Gastroenterol Nutr.* 1993;16:75-77

71. Nordstrom, E, Layde, P, Olson, K, et al. Roll-related occupational injuries on farms. *Am J Ind Med.* 1996 May;29(5):509-15

72. Martin S, Gordon T, Kupersmidt J. Survey of exposure to violence among the children of migrant and seasonal farm workers. *Public Health Rep.* 1995;110:268-276

73. Brindis C, Wolfe AL, McCarter V, Ball S, Starbuck-Morales S. The associations between immigrant status and risk-behavior patterns in Latino adolescents. *J Adolesc Health.* 1995;17:99-105

74. Wolfenden K, McKenzie A, Sanson-Fisher R. Identifying hazards and risk opportunity in child farm injury. *Aust J Public Health.* 1992;16:122-128

75. Esposito T, Sanddal ND, Dean JM, Hansen JD, Reynolds SA, Batlan K. Analysis of preventable trauma deaths and inappropriate trauma care in a rural state. *J Trauma.* 1995;39:955-962

76. Wright K. Management of agricultural injuries and illness. *Rural Nursing* 1993;28:253-266

77. Freudenberg K. The migrant farmworker: health care challenge. *N J Med.* 1992;89:581-585

78. Ciesielski SD, Seed JR, Esposito DH, Hunter N. The epidemiology of tuberculosis among North Carolina migrant farmworkers. *JAMA.* 1991;265:1715-1719

79. Richard JR. TB in migrant farmworkers. *JAMA.* 1994;271:905-906

80. Garcia JG, Matheny Dresser KS, Zerr AD. Respiratory health of Hispanic migrant farmworkers in Indiana. *Am J Ind Med.* 1996;29:23-32

81. HIV infection, syphilis, and tuberculosis screening among migrant farm workers—Florida, 1992. *MMWR Morb Mortal Wkly Rep.* 1992;41:723-725

82. Starke JR, Correa AG. Management of mycobacterial infection and disease in children. *Pediatr Infect Dis J.* 1995;14:455-469, quiz 469-470

83. American Academy of Pediatrics. Tuberculosis. In: Pickering LK, ed. *2000 Red Book: Report of the Committee on Infectious Diseases.* 25th ed. Elk Grove Village, Ill: American Academy of Pediatrics, 2000:593-613

84. Ciesielski SD, Seed JR, Ortiz JC, Metts J. Intestinal parasites among North Carolina migrant farm workers. *Am J Public Health.* 1992;82:1258-1262

85. Kirchoff LV. American trypanosomiasis (Chagas' disease)— a tropical disease now in the United States. Review. *N Engl J Med.* 1993;329:639-644

86. Maldonado YA, Nahlen BL, Roberto RR, et al. Transmission of plasmodium vivax malaria in San Diego County, California, 1986. *Am J Trop Med Hyg.* 1990;42:3-9

87. Singal M, Shaw PK, Lindsay RC, Roberto RR. An outbreak of introduced malaria in California possibly involving secondary transmission. *Am J Trop Med Hyg.* 1977;26:1-9

88. Anonymous. HIV risk 10 times higher for migrant farm workers. *Public Health Rep.* 1994;109:459

89. Centers for Disease Control and Prevention (CDC). HIV seroprevalence in migrant and seasonal farmworkers, North Carolina, 1987. *MMWR Morb Montal Wkly Rep.* 1988;37:517-519

90. HIV infection, syphilis, and tuberculosis screening among migrant farmworkers — Florida, 1992. *MMWR Morb Mortal Wkly Rep.* 1992;41:723-725

91. Lafferty J. Self-injection and needle sharing among migrant farm workers. *Am J Public Health.* 1991;81:221

92. HIV infection, syphilis, and tuberculosis screening among migrant farm workers — Florida, 1992. *MMWR Morb Mortal Wkly Rep.* 1992;41:723-725

93. Neill MA, Hightower AW, Broome CV. Leprosy in the United States, 1971-1981. *J Infect Dis.* 1985;152:1064-1069

Resources

Well-Child Visits

American Academy of Pediatrics. *Clinicians Handbook
of Preventive Services: Put Prevention Into Practice.*
Elk Grove Village, Ill: American Academy of Pediatrics;
1994

American Academy of Pediatrics Ad Hoc Task Force on
Definition of the Medical Home. The medical home.
Pediatrics. 1992;90:774

American Academy of Pediatrics Committee on Psychological
Aspects of Child and Family Health. *Guidelines for Health
Supervision III.* Elk Grove Village, Ill: American Academy
of Pediatrics; 1997

American Academy of Pediatrics Committee on Practice and
Ambulatory Medicine. Recommendations for preventive
pediatric health care. *Pediatrics.* 2000;105:645-646

Buirski N. *Earth angels: Migrant children in America.* San
Francisco, Calif: Pomegranate Artbooks; 1994

Frankenburg WK, Dodds J, Archer P, et al. *Denver II.* Denver,
Colo: Denver Developmental Materials; 1990

Frankenburg WK, Lynch K, White W, Brayden RM. The
"Partners" program: a prescription for preventive care.
Contemp Pediatr. 1996;13:65-70

Green M. Tasks of the times. *Contemp Pediatr.* 1996;13:94-104

Michael RJ, Salend SJ. Health problems of migrant children.
J Sch Health. 1985;55:411-412

Schneider B. Providing for the health needs of migrant children.
Nurse Pract. 1986;11:54-65

Special report: Clinical preventive services. What's really worth
doing for children. *Contemp Pediatr.* 1996;13:106-108, 113

National Center for Education in Maternal and Child Health
2000 15th St N, Suite 701
Arlington, VA 22201
Telephone: 703/524-7802
Fax: 703/524-9335
E-mail: brightfutures@ncemch.org
Web site: http://www.brightfutures.org
  Produces the book:
  Green M, Palfrey JS, eds. *Bright Futures: Guidelines for Health Supervision of Infants, Children, and Adolescents, 2nd ed.* Arlington, Va: National Center for Education in Maternal and Child Health, 2000

National Center for Farmworker Health, Inc.
PO Box 15009
Austin, TX 78715
Telephone: 512/312-2700
Fax: 512/312-2600
Web site: http://www.ncfh.org
  Produces the publication *Orientation to Multicultural Health Care in Migrant Health Programs.*

Reach Out and Read National Center
Boston Medical Center, One BMC Place
5th Floor High Rise
Boston, MA 02118
Telephone: 617/414-5701
Fax: 617/414-7557
E-mail: ror@bmc.org
Web site: http://www.bmc.org
  The Reach Out and Read pediatric early literacy program can help pediatricians make literacy part of pediatric primary care.

School Readiness

Children's Television Workshop Health and Safety Outreach
PO Box 55742
Indianapolis, IN 46205
Web site: http://www.sesamestreet.com

Produces the kit "Sesame Street Beginnings: Language to Literacy." The kit shows parents and caregivers how to take advantage of the daily opportunities to help children develop language skills and a love of books. Each kit includes a video; an audiocassette; a poster promoting daily routines that help develop language; a set of book-plates; Parent Pages that show adults fun activities that develop language skills; and a Facilitator Guide to help professionals use the materials. All materials are in English and Spanish. The kit can be ordered by sending a check or money order for $35 payable to Children's Television Workshop to the address above.

National Association for the Education of Young Children (NAEYC)
1509 16th St NW
Washington, DC 20036-1426
Telephone: 202/232-8777
   or 800/ 424-2460
Fax: 202/328-1846
E-mail: naeyc@naeyc.org
Web site: http://www.naeyc.org

National Child Care Information Center
301 Maple Ave W, Suite 602
Vienna, VA 22180
Telephone: 800/616-2242
Web site: http://www.ncic.org

National Education Goals Panel
1255 22nd St NW, Suite 502
Washington, DC 20037
Telephone: 202/724-0015
Fax: 202/632-0957
E-mail: negp@ed.gov
Web site: http://www.negp.gov

Immunizations

See also the **Vaccines for Children** section in Chapter 5
and the **Infectious Diseases** resources on page 136.

American Academy of Pediatrics
Division of Marketing and Publications
141 Northwest Point Blvd
Elk Grove Village, IL 60007
Telephone: 800/433-9016
Web site: http://www.aap.org
   Produces the *Before It's Too Late, Vaccinate* video and
   other immunization materials.

Adolescent Care

American Academy of Pediatrics Committee on Community
   Health Services. Health care for children of farmworker
   families. *Pediatrics.* 1995;95:952-953

Kleinman A, Eisenberg L, Good B. Culture, illness and care:
   clinical lessons from anthropological and cross-cultural
   research. *Ann Intern Med.* 1978;88:251-258

Manaster GJ, Chan JC, Safady R. Mexican-American migrant
   students' academic success: sociological and psychological
   acculturation. *Adolescence.* 1992;27:123-136

Tripp-Reimer T, Brink PJ, Saunders JM. Cultural assessment:
   context and process. *Nurs Outlook.* 1984;32:78-82

Oral Health

American Academy of Pediatric Dentistry (AAPD)
211 E Chicago Ave, #700
Chicago, IL 60611
Telephone: 312/337-2169
Fax: 312/337-6329

American Dental Association (ADA)
211 E Chicago Ave
Chicago, IL 60611
Telephone: 312/440-2500 or 800/947-4746 (product catalog)
Fax: 312/440-2800
Web site: http://www.ada.org/p&s/history/contact.html
    The ADA has excellent patient education materials in
    a variety of languages

National Institute of Dental Research
PO Box 54793
Washington, DC 20032
Telephone: 301/496-4261
    Provides the free brochure: *A Healthy Mouth For Your Baby*
    in English and Spanish.

National Oral Health Information Clearinghouse
1 NOHIC Way
Bethesda, MD 20892
Telephone: 301/402-7364
Fax: 301/907-8830
E-mail: nidr@aerie.com
Web site: http://www.aerie.com/nohicweb/index.html
    This federal information clearinghouse has a variety of
    materials that can be ordered in bulk. Some materials
    are free.

University of Washington, School of Dentistry
Box 357137
Seattle, WA 98195
Telephone: 206/543-5448
Fax: 206/543-6465
E-mail: uwcde@u.washington.edu
Web site: http://www.dental.washington.edu/pedo/edu.htm
The following package of resources can be purchased individually or together from the school's Continuing Education Department:

- Video — *Baby Teeth: Love 'em, Lose 'em* (English/Spanish). This excellent and entertaining video teaches parents how to care for infants' and toddlers' teeth.

- Video — *Lift the Lip: How to Check Infant and Toddler Teeth* (English/Spanish). This well-designed and very useful video teaches parents and non-dental professionals how to screen an infant and young toddler for pre-decay lesions and decayed teeth.

- *Lift the Lip Flip Chart: How to Check Infant and Toddler Teeth.* This flip chart is designed to enhance in-office oral health education by raising parental awareness. It explains to parents how to examine their child's teeth and what to look for.

Environmental Concerns

Please note that most local health departments have a lead poisoning coordinator.

American Academy of Pediatrics Committee on Environmental Health. *Handbook of Pediatric Environmental Health.* Elk Grove Village, Ill: American Academy of Pediatrics; 1999

Haddad LM, Shannon MW, Winchester JF, Winchester JP. *Clinical Management of Poisoning and Drug Overdose* 3rd ed. Philadelphia, Pa: WB Saunders; 1998.

Jackson RJ. The hazards of pesticides to children. In: Brooks SM, Gochfeld M, Herzstein J, Jackson RJ, Schenker MB, *Environmental Medicine.* St Louis, Mo: Mosby; 1995:377-382

Lessenger J, Estock M, Younglove T. An analysis of 190 cases of suspected pesticide illness. *J Am Board Fam Pract.* 1995;8:278-282

Morgan D, Reigart JR, Roberts JR, eds. *Recognition and Management of Pesticide Poisonings,* 5th ed. Washington, DC: US Environmental Protection Agency; 1999

O'Malley M. Clinical evaluation of pesticide exposure and poisonings. Review. *Lancet.* 1997;349:1161-1166

Reigart JR. Pesticides and children. *Pediatr Ann.* 1995;24:663-668

Rodgers GC Jr, Matyunas NJ. *Handbook of Common Poisonings in Children,* 3rd ed. Elk Grove Village, Ill: American Academy of Pediatrics; 1994

Schuman SH, Simpson WM Jr. *Ag-med: The Rural Practitioner's Guide to Agromedicine: Diagnosis and Management at a Glance.* Kansas City, Mo: National Rural Health Association; 1998

Wagner S, ed. Cholinesterase-inhibiting pesticide toxicity. In: *Case Studies in Environmental Medicine.* Vol 22. Atlanta, Ga: Agency for Toxic Substances and Disease Registry; 1993

Zwiener R, Ginsberg C. Organophosphate and carbamate poisoning in infants and children. *Pediatrics.* 1988;81: 121-126

Environmental and Occupational Health Sciences Institute
170 Frelinghuysen Rd
Piscataway, NJ 08854
Telephone: 732/445-0200
Fax: 732/445-0122
E-mail: rc@eohsi.rutgers.edu
Web site: http://www.eohsi.rutgers.edu/rc/publication.html
   Produces brochures on a wide variety of environmental and occupational health sciences topics in clear, everyday language.

Extoxnet

Web site: http://ace.orst.edu/info/extoxnet/

This pesticides information program is run by Cornell University, Oregon State University, and Michigan State University. Internet files on pesticides including trade names, regulatory status, acute and chronic toxicity, reproductive, and ecological effects are maintained on this site. The files are updated and contain extensive references.

National Center for Environmental Health

Centers for Disease Control and Prevention, Mail Stop F-29

4770 Buford Hwy NE

Atlanta, GA 30341-3724

Telephone: 770/488-7000, emergency response, 770/488-7100

E-mail: ncehinfo@cdc.gov

This is the designated national resource center for childhood lead poisoning.

National Center for Environmental Publications and Information

PO Box 42419

Cincinnati, OH 45242-2419

Telephone: 513/489-8190 or 800/490-9198

Fax: 513/489-8695

The Center provides free US Environmental Protection Agency pamphlets including, "Our Citizen's Guide to Pest Control and Pesticide Safety," "Pest Control in the School Environment," "Healthy Lawn, Healthy Environment," and fact sheets on lawn care, pesticide labels, and pesticide safety.

National Pesticide Telecommunications Network/Oregon State University

333 Weniger Hall
Corvallis, OR 97331-6502
Telephone: 800/858-7377 (for health professionals)
Web site: http://ace.orst.edu/info/nptn/

Provides excellent, free technical information on pesticides.

National Safety Council

1121 Spring Lake Dr
Itasca, IL 60143-3201
Telephone: 630/285-1121,
Lead information number: 800/424-LEAD (5323)
Fax: 630/285-1315
Web site: http://www.nsc.org/

The council cosponsors the "Sesame Street Lead Away!" project. Call for audiocassettes, comic booklets, videos, and posters. The audiotapes and comic books are in English and Spanish, and many of the materials are free.

Northwest Coalition for Alternatives to Pesticides

PO Box 1393
Eugene, OR 97440
Telephone: 541/344-5044
Fax: 541/344-6923
E-mail: info@pesticide.org

The coalition provides pamphlets on least toxic and alternatives to pesticides for the management of pest problems.

Child Maltreatment

Briere J, Berliner L, Bulkey JA, Jenny C, Reid T, eds. *The APSAC Handbook on Child Maltreatment.* Thousand Oaks, Calif: Sage; 1996

Echeverry JJ. Treatment barriers: accessing and accepting professional help. In Garcia JG, Zea MC, eds. *Psychological Interventions and Research With Latino Populations.* Boston, Mass: Allyn and Bacon; 1997

Garbarino J, Ebata A. The significance of ethnic and cultural differences in child maltreatment. *J Marriage Fam.* 1983;45:733-783

Hu T, Snowden LR, Jerrel JM. Costs and use of public mental health services by ethnicity. *J Ment Health Admin.* 1992;19:278-287

Korbin J, ed. *Child Abuse and Neglect: Cross-Cultural Perspectives.* Berkeley, Calif: University of California Press; 1981

Koss-Chioino JD. Traditional and folk approaches among ethnic minorities. In: Aponte JF, Rivers RY, Wohl J, eds. *Psychological Interventions and Cultural Diversity.* Boston, Mass; Allyn and Bacon; 1995:145-163

Pinderhughes EB. Empowerment for our clients and for ourselves. *Soc Casework.* 1983;64:331-338

Sue DW, Sue D. *Counseling the Culturally Different: Theory and Practice.* New York, NY: Wiley; 1990

American Professional Society on the Abuse of Children
407 S Dearborn, #1300
Chicago, IL 60605
Telephone: 312/554-0166
Fax: 312/554-0919
Web site: http://www.apsac.org

Child Welfare League of America
440 First St, NW, Suite 310
Washington, DC 20001-2085
Telephone: 202/638-2952
Fax: 202/638-4004
Web site: http://www.cwla.org

International Society for the Prevention of Child Abuse and Neglect
401 N Michigan Ave, Suite 2200
Chicago, IL 60611
Telephone: 312/644-4410
Fax: 312/321-6869
E-mail: kim_svevo@sba.com
Web site: http://ispcan.org

National Center for Missing and Exploited Children
2101 Wilson Blvd, Suite 550
Arlington, VA 22201
Telephone: 703/235-3900 or 800/843-5678
Web site: http://www.missingkids.org/

National Children's Advocacy Center
200 Westside Square, Suite 700
Huntsville, AL 35801
Telephone: 256/533-0531
Fax: 256/534-6883
E-mail: webmaster@ncac-hsv.org
Web site: http://www.ncac-hsv.org/

**National Clearinghouse on Child Abuse
and Neglect Information**
330 C Street SW
Washington, DC 20447
Telephone: 800/394-3366 or 703/385-7565
Fax: 703/385-3206
E-mail: nccanch@calib.com
Web site: http://www.calib.com/nccanch

National Network of Children's Advocacy Centers
1319 F Street NW, Suite 1001
Washington, DC 20004-1106
Telephone: 202/639-0597 or 800/239-9950
E-mail: info@nncac.org
Web site: http://www.nncac.org

National Organization for Parents Anonymous
675 W Foothill Blvd, Suite 220
Claremont, CA 91711-3475
Telephone: 909/621-6184
Fax: 909/625-6304
Web site: http://www.parentsanonymous-natl.org

**Parents United/Daughters and Sons United/
Adults Molested as Children United**
232 E Gish Rd, 1st Floor
San Jose, CA 95112
Telephone: 408/453-7616
E-mail: SJPU@Localink.net

Injuries

National Committee on Child Agriculture Injuries. *Children and Agriculture: Opportunities for Safety and Health.* National Committee on Child Agriculture Injuries; 1996

National Children's Center for Rural and Agricultural Health and Safety
1000 North Oak Ave
Marshfield, WI 54449
Telephone: 888/924-SAFE (7233)
Fax: 715/389-4996
Web site: http://research.marshfieldclinic.org/children/
Through the center, you can order *The North American Guidelines for Children's Agricultural Tasks.*

Infectious Diseases

1997 USPHS/JDSA report on the prevention of opportunistic infections in patients infected with human immunodeficiency virus. *Pediatrics.* 1998;102(suppl):1064-1086
American Academy of Pediatrics. *2000 Red Book: Report of the Committee on Infectious Diseases.* 25th ed. Elk Grove Village, Ill: American Academy of Pediatrics; 2000
American Academy of Pediatrics Committee on Pediatric AIDS. Evaluation and medical treatment of the HIV-exposed infant. *Pediatrics.* 1997;99:909-917
Antiretroviral Therapy and Medical Management of Pediatric HIV infection. *Pediatrics.* 1998;102(suppl):1005-1062
Correa A. Congenital syphilis: evaluation, diagnosis, and treatment. *Sem Pediatr Infect Dis.* 1994;5:30-34
Drugs for parasitic infections. *Med Lett.* 1995;40:99-108
Occupational Safety and Health Administration: Field Sanitation. *Federal Register.* 1987;52:16050-16068
Ussery XT, Valway SE, McKenna M, et al. Epidemiology of tuberculosis among children in the United States: 1985-1994. *Pediatr Infect Dis J.* 1996;15:697-704

Centers for Disease Control and Prevention

Web site: http://www.cdc.gov

Malaria Hotline	800/311-3435
National AIDS Hotline	800/342-2437
National HIV/AIDS Hotline (Spanish)	800/344-7432
National Immunization Hotline (English)	800/232-2522
National Immunization Hotline (Spanish)	800/232-0233
National STD Hotline	800/227-8922
Traveler's Health	877/394-8747
Tuberculosis Control	404/639-8120

National Hansen's Disease Program

1770 Physician Park Dr
Baton Rouge, LA 70816
Telephone: 800/642-2477

Provides consultation on clinical and pathologic issues related to leprosy/Hansen's Disease and can provide information about local leprosy clinics.

HIV/AIDS Treatment Information Service

PO Box 6303
Rockville, MD 20849-6303
Telephone: 800/448-0440

This is an information service for federally approved treatment guidelines and provides a bilingual reference specialist.

Leonard Wood Memorial American Leprosy Foundation

11600 Nebel St, #210
Rockville, MD 20852
Telephone: 301/984-1336

Maintains clinics and hospitals for diagnosis and treatment of leprosy.

Pediatric AIDS Clinical Trials Information Service
PO Box 6421
Rockville, MD 20849
Telephone: 800/Trials-A (874-2572)
> Provides information on therapeutic trials in HIV-infected children.

TB Net, Migrant Clinicians Network: The Binational Tuberculosis Tracking and Referral Project
PO Box 164285
Austin, TX 78716
Telephone: 800/825-8205
> This is a data transfer program for mobile populations with tuberculosis.

World Health Organization Action Programme for the Elimination of Leprosy
20 Avenue Appia CH-1211
Genève 27 Suisse
Web site: http://www.who.ch/programmes/lep/lep_home.htm
> Provides information regarding leprosy elimination programs in different countries.

Chapter 3: Programs and Organizations Related to Migrant Farmworkers

The following agencies below provide services and programs supporting migrant farmworkers and their families.

Farmworker Health Services, Inc
(formerly East Coast Migrant Health Project, Inc)
1234 Massachusetts Ave, NW
Washington, DC 20005
Telephone: 202/347-7377
Fax: 202/347-6385

>This agency works to assist farmworkers in accessing local services. It also assists local health agencies in improving their services for farmworkers.

Farmworker Justice Fund, Inc
1111 19th St, NW, Suite 1000
Washington, DC 20036
Telephone: 202/776-1757
Fax: 202/776-1792
E-mail: fjf@NCLR.org

>The Farmworker Justice Fund (FJF) is a private, nonprofit organization based in Washington, DC. This national advocacy organization works to improve the living and working conditions of migrant and seasonal farmworkers. Its primary functions include administrative agency monitoring, litigation, technical assistance, and public education. Each year, the FJF responds to requests for information, materials, and technical assistance from a variety of farmworker organizations, including migrant health centers, across the United States.

Migrant Clinicians Network, Inc
PO Box 164285
Austin, TX 78716
Telephone: 512/327-2017
Fax: 512/327-0719
E-mail: mcn@onr.com
Web site: http://www.migrantclinician.org

The Migrant Clinicians Network (MCN) is a network of more than 900 clinicians across the country and in Puerto Rico who serve migrant and seasonal farmworkers. The membership of the MCN is professionally diverse, including physicians, outreach workers, nurses, and other health professionals. The MCN mission is to promote the health of farmworkers. As a network, the MCN is a professional home for clinicians who serve migrant farmworkers that provides opportunities for networking and professional development; advances clinical effectiveness by conducting research and developing clinical tools; and acts as a national and international voice on migrant health issues through leadership, advocacy, and partnerships with collaborating agencies.

Migrant Education Program
Office of Migrant Education
US Department of Education
600 Independence Ave, SW
Room 4100 Portals Bldg
Washington, DC 20202-6153
Telephone: 800/234-8848 or 202/260-1164
Fax: 202/265-0089
Web site: http://www.ed.gov/offices/OESE/MEP

The Migrant Education Program provides supplemental education and support services to more than 600,000 children and youth nationwide. The program seeks to enable migrant children to meet the same student performance standards that are expected of all children by helping migrant children overcome the educational disruption, cultural and language barriers, social isolation, health problems, and other factors that may inhibit their ability to do well in school. Supportive health services could include medical, dental, nutritional, and psychological services that are provided in cooperation with other agencies.

Preschool and kindergarten programs designed to prepare migrant children for successful school experiences also are provided in areas where funding is available. These Migrant Education Preschool Programs are separate from other similar programs such as Head Start and Migrant Head Start. Children qualify for these different services based on each program's definition of "migrant."

To refer families to the Migrant Education Program or to get more information,

1. Contact your local school district to see if they have a Migrant Education Program. Ask for Title 1C or the Migrant Education Program coordinator.
2. Call the National Migrant Education Hotline, at 800/234-8848, which provides information and referrals related to education, health, housing, food, clothing, and emergencies.
3. Call your state Department of Education and ask for the federal programs coordinator. Find out who your state director of migrant education is, and request information relevant to services available in your community.

Migrant Head Start
330 C St SW
Washington, DC 20201
Telephone: 202/205-8455
Fax: 202/401-5916

> The Migrant Head Start Program was designed to ensure that migrant farmworker families have access to the full range of Head Start services. Services are identical for Migrant Head Start and Head Start, but migrant grantees modify delivery to meet the specific needs of farmworker

families. For example, some migrant centers provide extended child care services, usually 12 hours a day and 7 days a week during the height of the harvest season. In addition, Migrant Head Start serves infants, toddlers, and preschool children.

Migrant Health Program

Bureau of Primary Health Care
Health Resources and Services Administration
BPHC/DCMH/Migrant Health Branch
4350 East-West Hwy, 7th Floor
Bethesda, MD 20814
Telephone: 301/594-4303
Fax: 301/594-4997
Web site: http://www.bphc.hrsa.dhhs.gov/mhc/mhc1.htm

The Migrant Health Program is administered by the Bureau of Primary Health Care, in the Health Resources and Services Administration of the US Department of Health and Human Services. This program is a result of the 1962 Migrant Health Act, which authorizes the delivery of primary and supplemental health services to farmworkers. The program provides grant support to more than 120 community-based and state organizations to provide comprehensive primary care services that address the unique needs of migrant and seasonal farmworkers. An additional 600 community health centers are often included in the Migrant Health Program.

Migrant Health Promotion

(formerly Midwest Migrant Health Information Office)
502 W Elm Ave
Monroe, MI 48162
Telephone: 734/243-0711
Fax: 734/243-0435
E-mail: mhp@tdi.net
Web site: http://monroe.lib.mi.us/cwis/migrheal.htm

Migrant Health Promotion (MHP) strives to enhance the health and well-being of farmworker families through collaborative peer education and advocacy programs designed to empower farmworkers. The MHP trains migrant farmworker men and women to be health promoters (Camp Health Aides and *Colonia* Health Workers). These health promoters provide peer health education, service information, translation, and basic first aid to isolated migrant camps. The MHP has established programs in Arizona, Florida, Illinois, Michigan, Minnesota, New Jersey, Ohio, Texas, and Wisconsin. The MHP provides technical assistance and distributes educational materials nationwide. The MHP also publishes a bilingual Migrant Health Services Directory.

National Advisory Council on Migrant Health
Bureau of Primary Health Care
Health Resources and Services Administration
BPHC/DCMH/Migrant Health Branch
4350 East-West Hwy, Room 7-5A1
Bethesda, MD 20814
Telephone: 301/594-4302
Fax: 301/594-4997
Web site: http://www.bphc.hrsa.dhhs.gov/mhc/mhc1.htm
    The National Advisory Council on Migrant Health is legislatively mandated to advise, consult with, and make recommendations to the US Department of Health and Human Services on the health and well-being of migrant farmworkers and their families. Recommendations from the 15-member council focus on access to health care, mental health, occupational safety and health, housing, and research. Council members are primarily farmworkers and former farmworkers. Public council meetings are held three times a year and input is sought through public hearings held annually. Transcripts of public testimony are provided on request.

National Association of Community Health Centers, Inc
1330 New Hampshire Ave NW, Suite 122
Washington, DC 20036
Telephone: 202/659-8008
Fax: 202/659-8519

This advocacy organization monitors federal policy and initiatives (including the implementation of the Immigration Bill) and participates in Migrant Health Branch work groups. It also coordinates farmworker health services by networking with other organizations that are active in the farmworker health arena.

National Center for Farmworker Health, Inc
1515 Capital of Texas Hwy S, Suite 220
Austin, TX 78746
Telephone: 512/328-7682
Fax: 512/328-8559
Web site: http://www.ncfh.org

The National Center for Farmworker Health works to improve the health status of farmworker families through the application of human, technical, and information resources. They conduct a variety of activities, including increasing public awareness of farmworker needs, increasing access to services by improving collaboration between organizations, enhancing the operation of health centers serving farmworkers, and operating a migrant information resource center.

National Immigration Law Center
1102 S Crenshaw Blvd, Suite 101
Los Angeles, CA 90019
Telephone: 213/938-6452
Fax: 213/964-7940
E-mail: hn0181@handsnet.org

The mission of the National Immigration Law Center (NILC) is to defend the rights of low-income immigrants. This support center provides advice, training, and litigation assistance to nonprofit agencies throughout the United States. The NILC also publishes several resource materials including a legal reference manual, a monthly law newsletter, a referral directory, and community education materials.

National Rural Health Association

One West Armour Blvd, Suite 301
Kansas City, MO 64111
Telephone: 816/756-3140
Fax: 816/756-3144
E-mail: mail@nrharural.org
Web site: http://www.NRHArural.org

The National Rural Health Association (NRHA) is a non-profit association composed of individual and organizational members who share a common interest in rural health. Its headquarters is in Kansas City, MO, and it has a government affairs office in Washington, DC. The mission of this organization is to improve the health and health care of rural Americans. The association provides a forum for the exchange and dissemination of ideas, information, research, and methods to improve rural health. The NRHA has an extensive list of publications and resources related to rural health issues.

Rural Community Assistance Program

602 S King St, Suite 402
Leesburg, VA 20175
Telephone: 703/771-8636
Fax: 703/771-8753
Web site: http://www.rcap.org

The mission of the Rural Community Assistance Program (RCAP) is to assist elected officials and residents of small, rural communities to improve their quality of life. Most RCAP projects are carried out in underserved rural areas with populations of 2,000 or less. The RCAP services are provided free of charge to these communities. The RCAP is a resource for community leaders and others looking for technical assistance services and training related to waste water treatment, solid waste programs, economic development, environmental health projects, and comprehensive community assessment and planning.

Chapter 4: Language Resources

Please note that this is not a comprehensive list and does not imply endorsement of these programs and resources. Also check your local bookstore or library to find a wide variety of books and tapes designed for professionals who have a limited amount of time.

Spanish Language

Medical Dictionary
Rogers GT. *English-Spanish Spanish-English Medical Dictionary.* New York, NY: McGraw-Hill, Inc, Health Professions Division; 1991

Self-study Guides
Tabery JJ, Webb MR, Mueller BV. *Communicating in Spanish for Medical Personnel.* Boston, Mass: Little, Brown; 1984
This self-study guide teaches users how to speak with patients at a basic level. It can be used as a guide for beginners or an improvement tool for those with some Spanish skills. The lessons are arranged according to a large variety of medical topics (admission to the hospital, prenatal care, etc).

Kelz RK. *Conversational Spanish for Medical Personnel, 2nd ed.* Albany, NY: Delmar Publishers Inc; 1982
This book includes written exercises for self-instruction as well as a dictionary of medical terminology.

Rajkovic AM. *Manual for (Relatively) Painless Medical Spanish: A Self-Teaching Course.* Austin, Tex: University of Texas Press; 1992
The easy-to-follow instructions in this manual teach the user how to put words and phrases together correctly. This is a very helpful guide for a beginner because most of the instructions are in English. This guide also includes a vocabulary of medical terms and appendices with phrases for adult history, pediatric history, physical exam, etc.

Joyce EV, Villanueva ME. *Say It In Spanish: A Guide for Health Care Professionals.* Philadelphia, Penn: WB Saunders; 1996
This conversation and phrase book also can be used as a self-instruction program. It includes some grammar instruction and many medical dialogue examples (physical exam, discharge planning, etc). The bilingual text on every page includes complete phrases with their Spanish translation and pronunciation guide. This book also includes a cultural perspective and information on home cures and popular beliefs.

Conversation and Phrase Books for Medical Personnel

Escandon R. *Bilingual Vocabulary for the Medical Profession.* Cincinnati, Ohio: Southwestern Publishing Co; 1982

Teed CA. *Conversational Spanish for the Medical and Health Professions.* New York, NY: Rinehart and Winston; 1983

Kelz RK. *Conversational Spanish for Medical Personnel: Essential Expressions, Questions, and Directions for Medical Personnel.* New York, NY: Wiley; 1982
This guide contains translations for common expressions, anatomical vocabulary, pronunciation guides, instruction on basic grammar, and a bilingual index. The guide also includes phrase translations for administrative personnel.

English and Spanish: Medical Words and Phrases. 2nd ed. Springhouse, Penn: Springhouse Corporation; 1999
This phrase book begins with some instruction on Spanish grammar and pronunciation, but the majority of the book includes Spanish translations for common medical dialogues. Health topics are arranged according to body systems with easy-to-locate sections. The book also includes an appendix with therapeutic drug classifications.

Wilber C J, Lister S. *Medical Spanish: The Instant Survival Guide.* Stoneham, Mass: Butterworth Publishers; 1983
Each section of this guide includes phrase translations for a variety of medical situations. There also is a section with patient education topics such as head injury observation,

care of burns, and cancer warning signs. This guide has helpful information on developing consent forms and other records and there are some translations for other medical personnel: dietitians, medical social workers, volunteers, and aide and homemaker services. The guide also includes a bilingual glossary, but no pronunciation guides.

Gonzalez-Lee T. *Medical Spanish: Interviewing the Latino Patient: A Cross-Cultural Perspective* (book and cassette). Englewood Cliffs, NJ: Prentice Hall; 1990

Kantrowitz MP, Mondragón A, Coleman WL. *¿Qué Pasó? An English-Spanish Guide for Medical Personnel.* Albuquerque, NM: University of New Mexico Press; 1983
This guide is easy to use and includes complete phrases for common medical situations. It has an extensive bilingual vocabulary section with common phrases and anatomical terms.

Harvey WC. *Spanish for Health Care Professionals.* Hauppauge, NY: Barron's Educational Series Inc; 1994
This guide has some basic information on communicating in Spanish followed by chapters with vocabulary and phrases for various medical topics (accidents, pregnancy, elderly patients, etc). This guide includes an extensive bilingual word and expression finder.

Machtinger E, Nigrovic PA. *Spanish for Pediatric Medicine: A Practical Communication Guide.* Elk Grove Village, Ill: American Academy of Pediatrics; 1997
This is a quick reference for identifying and exploring medical problems in well-child care, sick visits, and emergency settings. The guide takes into account the scheduled visits featured in *Guidelines for Health Supervision III.*

Spanish Phrases for Health Care Professionals. Rockville, Md: National Institutes of Health, Clinical Center Communications; 1988

Study Abroad/Intensive Learning Programs

AmeriSpan Unlimited

PO Box 40513
Philadelphia, PA 19106
Telephone: 800/879-6640 or 215/985-4522
Fax: 215/985-4524
E-mail: info@amerispan.com
Web site: http://www.amerispan.com

> This agency specializes in Spanish immersion and educational travel programs throughout Mexico, Central America, and South America. In addition to providing information on a large variety of schools available, this agency also acts as a travel agent to assist individuals with their travel plans. A wide variety of programs are available, ranging from beginners to those nearly fluent in Spanish. To learn medical Spanish, AmeriSpan suggests enrolling in private instruction courses at one of the better schools. Specific instruction in medical terms can be requested. The agency also offers medically related internship programs.

The Boston Language Institute

636 Beacon St
Boston, MA 02215
Telephone: 617/262-3500
Fax: 617/262-3595 or 617/247-3919
Web site: http://www.boslang.com

> The Boston Language Institute offers several programs of instruction (including medical Spanish) organized into different formats designed to meet your scheduling needs. The core program of 30 hours of instruction is approximately equivalent to one college semester of study. This core program is available in 10-week and accelerated 5-week sessions. The Boston Language Institute also offers intensive programs for students wishing to immerse themselves in a new language and a new culture in a short period of time.

Ghost Ranch Conference Center
Joe Keesecker, Director
HC 77, Box 11
Abiquiu, NM 87510
Telephone: 505/685-4333
E-mail: Joe.Keesecker@pcusa.org

A National Adult Study Center of the Presbyterian Church, this center offers a 2-week intensive Spanish course in the summer. The ranch is 120 miles from Albuquerque and serves as a year-round conference center for a variety of groups addressing concerns of church, society, and the arts.

Global Exchange
2017 Mission St, #303
San Francisco, CA 94110
Telephone: 415/255-7296

Global Exchange offers "Reality Tours" in many areas of the world, including Central America and the Caribbean. These alternative tours include visiting people's homes, government agencies, and activist groups. The trips last 2 weeks, and a flat fee includes all arrangements. Through this agency, stays at Mar de Jade in Nayarit, Mexico (on the Pacific coast), can be arranged. Mar de Jade offers rustic vacation accommodations as well as Spanish classes and volunteer opportunities in the nearby community clinic. Medical students, residents, registered nurses, and licensed vocational nurses may obtain university credit or continuing education units for this program.

Spanish Abroad, Inc

6520 N 41st St

Paradise Valley, AZ 85253

Telephone: 888/S-ABROAD or 602/947-4652

Fax: 602/840-1545

E-mail: info@spanishabroad.com

Web site: http://www.spanishabroad.com/

This agency provides information on a variety of language schools located throughout Latin America. It provides assistance in choosing the appropriate program and also can make arrangements to stay with local families. This agency suggests enrolling in a private instruction program to learn medical Spanish.

Studyabroad.com

Web site: http://www.studyabroad.com/studyabroad.com.html

This is an excellent online resource center. It provides information listings for thousands of study-abroad programs in more than 100 countries throughout the world, including intensive Spanish learning programs in Spain, Mexico, South America, Central America, and locations in the United States.

Learning on the Internet

PBS Adult Learning Service

Web site: http://www.pbs.org/teachersource/learn.shtm

Tecla

Web site: http://www.bbk.ac.uk/tecla/welcome.html

Tecla is a text magazine written for learners and teachers of Spanish. It is a joint production between the Spanish Department at Birkbeck College and the Consejería de Educación, Embajada de España en Londres. *Tecla* is written by Isabel Hernández Cánovas and Emma Nieves Trellez and edited by Rob Kennedy. It is produced weekly during the UK academic year.

Other Learning Opportunities

There are many opportunities to learn Spanish in individual communities. Look for Spanish or medical Spanish classes at

- Colleges and universities
- Public schools
- Special language schools
- Professional conferences or seminars that offer continuing education credit

Most colleges and universities now offer courses through a variety of methods, including correspondence classes, distance learning, telelearning, and online classes. Check the institutions in your area (most can provide excellent learning opportunities for professionals with a limited amount of time. Many universities and colleges have 1- or 2-week accelerated language programs in the summer.

Health Promotion/Patient Education Materials in Spanish

Substance Abuse and Mental Health Services Administration
Office of Communications and External Affairs
Parklawn Bldg, Room 13C05
5600 Fishers Ln
Rockville, MD 20857
Telephone: 301/443-8956 or 800/729-6686 (orders)
> Provides free educational materials on alcohol, drug abuse, and mental health

American Academy of Pediatrics
Division of Publications
PO Box 747
Elk Grove Village, IL 60009-0747
Telephone: 888/227-1770
Web site: http://www.aap.org/
> Has patient education brochures in Spanish

American Cancer Society

Telephone: 800/227-2345

> Has health promotion materials related to cancer and cancer prevention. Call the number listed above to find your local office.

American College of Obstetricians and Gynecologists

ACOG Distribution Center

PO Box 4500

Kearneysville, WV 25430-4500

Telephone: 304/725-8410 or 800/762-2264 (orders)

Fax: 800/525-5563

> Has patient education materials for contraception, pregnancy, labor and delivery, postpartum care, gynecologic problems, special procedures, and women's health

American Heart Association

Telephone: 800/AHA-USA1

> Has a wide variety of educational materials on heart disease and stroke. Call the number listed above to find your local office.

American Social Health Association

PO Box 13827

Research Triangle Park, NC 27709-3827

Telephone: 800/783-9877 (orders) or

919/361-8422 (customer service)

Fax: 919/361-8425

> Has educational materials on sexually transmitted diseases

Healthy Mothers, Healthy Babies Coalition

121 N Washington St, Suite 300

Alexandria, VA 22314

Telephone: 703/836-6110

Fax: 703/836-3470

> Has free educational materials on child and maternal health topics, provides information to health professionals

Migrant Health Promotion

502 W Elm Ave

Monroe, MI 48162

Telephone: 734/243-0711

Fax: 734/243-0435

E-mail: mhp@tdi.net

Web site: http://monroe.lib.mi.us/cwis/migrheal.htm

Has Spanish and bilingual training and educational materials including health manuals and flip charts

National AIDS Clearinghouse

Centers for Disease Control and Prevention (CDC)

PO Box 6003

Rockville, MD 20850

Telephone: 800/458-5231

Distributes publications on HIV/AIDS education. Materials are not free, but can be ordered in bulk.

National Cancer Institute

Office of Cancer Communications

Bldg 31, Room 10A24

9000 Rockville Pike

Bethesda, MD 20892

Telephone: 301/469-5583 or 800/422-6237 (orders)

Offers free health promotion materials on cancer and cancer prevention

National Clearinghouse for Alcohol and Drug Information

PO Box 2345

Rockville, MD 20847

Telephone: 301/468-2600 or 800/729-6686

Provides free educational materials on alcohol, tobacco, and other drugs

National Alliance for Hispanic Health
1501 Sixteenth St, NW
Washington DC 20036
Telephone: 202/387-5000
   Produces Spanish language health materials and serves as
   a resource for information about other resources

National Diabetes Information Clearinghouse
1 Information Way
Bethesda, MD 20892-3560
Telephone: 301/654-3327
   Provides free educational materials on diabetes and related
   complications

National Digestive Disease Information Clearinghouse
2 Information Way
Bethesda, MD 20892-3570
Telephone: 301/654-3810
   Distributes free educational materials on digestive health

National Institutes of Health
Division of Public Information
9000 Rockville Pike
Bldg 31, Room 2B-10
Bethesda, MD 20892
Telephone: 301/496-1766
   Provides free educational materials on a variety of health
   topics

National Institute of Mental Health
The Parklawn Bldg
5600 Fishers Ln 7C-02
Rockville, MD 20857
Telephone: 301/443-4513
Fax: 301/443-0008
> Provides free educational materials on a wide variety of
> mental health topics

National Institute for Occupational Safety and Health
Technical Information Branch
4676 Columbia Pkwy
Cincinnati, OH 45226
Telephone: 800/356-4674
> Provides a limited number of free educational materials
> on workplace safety

National Lead Safety Council
Telephone: 800/424-LEAD(5323)
Fax: 202/659-1192
E-mail: ehc@cais.com
> Produces and distributes the "Sesame Street Lead Away"
> materials — audio cassettes, videos, comic booklets,
> posters — in English and Spanish. Many materials are free.
> Videos are in English only. Also check with your local PBS
> station; the station may have copies for free distribution.

National Safety Council
1121 Springlake Dr
Itasca, IL 60143-3201
Telephone: 630/285-1121
> Provides educational materials related to accident prevention
> and safety

Texas Department of Health
Materials Acquisition and Management Division
Attn: Warehouse Manager
1100 W 49th St
Austin, TX 78756
Telephone: 512/458-7111
> Has health promotion and patient education materials for
> a variety of topics. Also check your local or state health
> department for Spanish materials.

Haitian Creole Language

There are limited resources for learning the Haitian Creole
language, for this reason sources are listed for some of the
texts. Check these sources for other titles as well. Another
resource is your local bookstore or library. Note that Haitian
Creole is also spelled Haitian-Kreol or Kreyòl.

Dictionaries
Teodore C. *Creole-English English-Creole Dictionary.* New
York, NY: Hippocrene Books; 1995
> This is a basic dictionary and does not include phrases,
> pronunciation guides, or other explanations, but it is
> comprehensive and concise.

Freeman BC. *Haitian Creole-English/ English-Haitian Creole
Medical Dictionary, with Glossary of Food and Drink:
Medicine In Haiti II.* Port-au-Prince: La Presse Evangelique;
Lawrence, Kansas: University of Kansas, 1992

Self-study Guides

Valdman, A. *Ann Pale Kreyól: An Introductory Course in Haitian Creole*. Bloomington, Ind: Creole Insitute, Indiana University; 1988

This title is available from:
The Creole Institute
Ballantine Hall 604
Indiana University
Bloomington, IN 47405
Telephone: 812/855-4988
Fax: 812/855-2386
Web site: http://php.indiana.edu/~valdman/home.html

Savain RE. *Haitian-Kreol In Ten Steps*. Rochester, Vt: Schenkman Books, Inc; 1993

This is a good primer on Haitian-Kreol and includes the alphabet, pronunciation, and grammatical rules. This book is user-friendly in its workbook-style layout. There is a sample form in the back of the book (name, date, other demographic and personal information).

Language Tapes

Basic Haitian Creole
Includes 15.5 hours of tapes, 24 lessons, and a textbook with glossaries.

Let's Speak Creole
Includes a 25-chapter text, readings, and 12 hours of tapes.

Pimsleur Haitian Creole
Includes 5 hours of tapes.

The above tapes are available from
World of Reading, Ltd
PO Box 13092
Atlanta, GA 30324-0092
Telephone: 404/233-4042 or 800/729-3703
Fax: 404/237-5511
E-mail: Polyglot@wor.com
Web site: http://www.wor.com

Freeman, B. *Survival Creole.*

Freeman, B. Ti Koze Kreyòl: *A Haitian-Creole Conversation Manual*

The above tapes are available from
Mount Oread Bookshop, The Kansas Union
Jayhawk Blvd
The University of Kansas
Lawrence, KS 66045
Telephone: 800/458-1111
E-mail: oread@union.wpo.ukans.edu
Web site: http://www.jayhawks.com/oread/index.html

Study Abroad

The Boston Language Institute

See the description in the Study Abroad/Intensive Learning Programs section.

Global Exchange

See the description in the Study Abroad/Intensive Learning Programs section.

Chapter 5: Policies Affecting Migrant Farmworkers' Children

Fair Labor Standards Act

There are few laws regulating child labor on farms. The Fair Labor Standards Act of 1974 (FLSA), for example, has few protections for children involved in agricultural labor.[1] This legislation establishes age 12 as the minimum age for farm work but creates exemptions for children as young as 10 years of age.[2] Older children can work for unlimited hours, and those 16 years of age are allowed to perform hazardous jobs in farm labor.[3] The FLSA language states that children 14 to 16 years old working in agriculture (something other than manufacturing or mining) does not constitute "oppressive child labor" so long as such employment does not interfere with their education or with their health.[1]

The FLSA does contain provisions that authorize the US Secretary of Labor to investigate and inspect a workplace with respect to the employment of minors.[4] The Secretary of Labor also is authorized to ask the attorney general to bring an action against an employer to enjoin the practice of "oppressive child labor."[5] The secretary may require that employers obtain proof of age from an employee.[6]

One of the problems with child labor protective legislation is the government's capacity for monitoring and enforcement of these regulations. Few agencies, including the Department of Labor (DOL), have the manpower and financial resources to investigate each and every farm where migrant and seasonal farmworkers may work along with their minor children. Currently, the DOL has about 1,000 investigators looking for farm workplace violations[7] in this country, where it is estimated that there are 800,000 farms that hire labor.[8] The US General Accounting Office reports a significant number of injuries and deaths due to violations of child labor laws.[2] The AFOP

Washington *Newsline,* published by the Association of Farm-worker Opportunity Programs, reports that more than 3 million children work in the United States, and about 500 are injured daily.[7] Once an injury occurs due to a violation of the FLSA, all that the Secretary of Labor can do is to fine the employers and hope that this step is sufficient to stop "oppressive child labor" practices and prevent future injuries at that farm.

Migrant Health Programs

The Migrant Health Act was signed into law in 1962 during the Kennedy administration to authorize the delivery of primary and supplemental health services to migrant and seasonal farmworkers.[9] The Migrant Health Program was to be administered by the US Department of Health and Human Services, and its purpose was to provide health care services to migrant farmworkers and their families.

While there are more than 100 centers across the country currently funded by the Migrant Health Act, studies have shown that these centers only are able to serve about 15% of the migrant population due to lack of resources and limited funding.[9] These centers have autonomy over the care provided, and there is no directive or specific funding that focuses on the needs of children.

1. **Who is eligible to receive care at these migrant health care centers?**

   To be eligible for care at a migrant health care center under the Migrant Health Act, a person must fall under one of the following categories:

   a. Migratory agricultural worker: An individual whose principal employment is in agriculture on a seasonal basis...and who establishes for the purposes of such employment a temporary abode.[10]

   b. Seasonal agricultural worker: An individual whose principal employment is in agriculture on a seasonal basis and who is not a migratory agricultural worker.[11]

However, according to the Migrant Health Act, a migrant health center is one that provides patient case management services "for migrant agricultural workers, seasonal agricultural workers, and the members of the families of such migratory and seasonal workers, within the area it serves... ."[12]

2. How long is a person eligible for health care at these centers?

A person is eligible for care at a migrant health care center so long as that person "has been so employed within the last 24 months"[10] or has previously met the definition of a migratory agricultural worker under 42 USC §254b(a)(2) but can no longer meet that definition "because of age or disability."[12] Therefore, children are eligible for these services so long as their parents fall under this definition.

Medicaid

The Medicaid program was created by the federal government in 1965 in an effort to provide health care to people with low income.[13] Beneficiaries of this entitlement program are generally low-income pregnant women and children and individuals who are aged, blind, or disabled, although the specific requirements vary state by state. In 1999, one in five children were insured by Medicaid.[14] This program is coordinated by the federal, state, and local governments and is generally administered by the state governments through welfare departments. The federal government pays for most of the cost of Medicaid and that percentage varies in each state according to the number of low-income people living in that state.[13] Eligibility and coverage for Medicaid does vary in each state but there are some basic federal requirements for eligibility that must be met by all state programs. Changes in welfare legislation in 1996 altered eligibility requirements as well. These federal requirements have been changed over the years, most recently by legislation in 1996 and the Balanced Budget Act of 1997.

1. Who is eligible for Medicaid?

The purpose of the Medicaid program has been to provide health coverage for low-income people, traditionally those receiving cash welfare benefits through Aid to Families with Dependent Children (AFDC) and those who are aged, blind, or disabled receiving cash benefits under the Supplemental Security Income (SSI). Medicaid eligibility was based on AFDC rules determining how to categorize income and resources. The same AFDC criteria was used in those states with "medically needy programs" to determine eligibility.[15] The Personal Responsibility and Work Opportunity Reconciliation Act of 1996 (PL 104-193) de-linked the Medicaid program from cash assistance programs. The federal requirements for Medicaid coverage under the new law are

- Pregnant women, children, and caretakers of children who would have been eligible for Medicaid under the AFDC rules before July 16, 1996, regardless of whether they actually received AFDC cash benefits before that time.[15]

- Those receiving SSI, or in states using more restrictive criteria, those aged, blind and disabled individuals who meet criteria more restrictive than that of the SSI program.[16]

- Infants born to Medicaid-eligible pregnant women for the first year of life.[16]

- Children younger than age 6 and pregnant women who meet the state's AFDC financial requirements or whose family income is at or below 133% of the federal poverty level. States are required to extend Medicaid eligibility until age 19 to all children born after September 30, 1983, in families with incomes at or below the federal poverty level.[16]

- Adoption assistance and foster care assistance recipients under Title IV-E of the Social Security Act.[16]

- Special protected groups who lose cash assistance because of the cash programs' rules but who may keep Medicaid for a period of time.[16]

The new laws allow states to change AFDC rules in effect as of July 16, 1996, for Medicaid eligibility purposes. Transitional Medicaid also has been extended until the year 2001 for those families who suddenly do not qualify for cash benefits because of "socially desirable reasons," such as those with a higher income due to employment or due to child support collections who continue to have a need for Medicaid during a transition period. Recipients who lose cash benefits under the new law may lose Medicaid if they refuse to work. The states are allowed to deny cash benefits to an entire family for violation of the work provision, but Medicaid may not be denied to minor children under this provision.[15]

The Balanced Budget Act contains three additional provisions that are designed to increase coverage for children. These provisions give states the option to establish coverage under the following principles: (1) presumptive eligibility for children, (2) coverage of children receiving SSI and (3) the option to provide 12-month continuous coverage.[17] Thus, the states can facilitate the enrollment of children by establishing presumptive Medicaid eligibility for children by continuing coverage for all disabled children who were receiving SSI on August 22, 1996; and by guaranteeing 12 months of coverage to children enrolled in Medicaid regardless of whether the children experienced changes in family income or other circumstances that would make them ineligible for Medicaid during that period of time.[17]

2. **What is the relationship between eligibility and citizenship?**
Following the Personal Responsibility and Work Opportunity Reconciliation Act of 1996, individuals who meet the eligibility requirements of Medicaid but are not citizens or nationals

of the United States can only receive Medicaid under certain conditions. Medicaid must be provided to eligible citizens or nationals of the United States. Individuals who are not citizens or nationals of the United States only are eligible to receive treatment for emergency medical conditions. The new law only distinguishes between qualified or non-qualified aliens for purposes of Medicaid coverage.[18] The distinctions are listed in Table 5.1 and are generally applicable to all federal programs with few exceptions. States have the option to bar or limit access to Temporay Assistance for Needy Families (TANF), Title XX state-funded benefit programs.

3. **Will aliens receiving Medicaid benefits or SSI before August 22, 1996, lose their benefits?**
   States must continue to provide Medicaid to any person who was lawfully residing in that state, who continues to meet the state's Medicaid eligibility criteria, and who was receiving Medicaid on August 22, 1996, but was not receiving SSI before January 1, 1997.[18] This requirement applies to the individual regardless of age.

   States also must continue to provide Medicaid to aliens receiving SSI before August 22, 1996. Those receiving SSI with "questionable or unknown citizenship status" will be sent notices to provide the necessary proof so that payments can continue.[18] Again, this requirement applies to the individual regardless of age.

4. **What care can eligible non-qualified aliens receive under Medicaid?**
   Those who are non-qualified aliens but who meet other Medicaid eligibility standards are eligible for Medicaid only for treatment of emergency medical conditions.[18] To be eligible for these services, an alien must meet all the eligibility requirements for Medicaid under that state's particular plan. Care and services must be necessary for the

Immigration Status	Eligibility for Medicaid if Admitted to the United States Before 8/22/96	Eligibility for Medicaid if Admitted to the United States On or After 8/22/96	Eligibility for Emergency Medicaid
	Table 5-1 **Conditions for Medicaid Eligibility[18]**		
US citizen	Yes	Yes	Yes
Legal permanent resident except Amerasian legal permanent residents	Yes	Not eligible for the first 5 years in the United States, except • An honorably discharged veteran or active duty military member • A spouse, unmarried surviving spouse, or un-married minor child of an honorably discharged veteran or active duty military member	Yes
Amerasian legal permanent resident	Yes	Yes, for the first 5 years after the legal date of entry	Yes
Refugee under §207 Immigration and Naturalization Act	Yes	Yes, for the first 7 years after the legal date of entry	Yes
Asylee under §208 Immigration and Naturalization Act			
Alien whose deportation is withheld under §242(h) or §241(b)(3) Immigration and Naturalization Act			
Cuban or Haitian entrant paroled under §212(d)(5) Immigration and Naturalization Act			
Parolee (other than Cuban and Haitian entrant) under §212(5)(d) Immigration and Naturalization Act	Yes	No	Yes
Conditional entrant under §203(a)(7) Immigration and Naturalization Act	Yes	No	Yes
Non-qualified alien	No	No	No
Nonimmigrant alien			
Undocumented alien			

treatment of an emergency medical condition. Care and services cannot be related to either an organ transplant procedure or routine prenatal or postpartum care. The medical condition (including emergency labor and delivery) has to have symptoms with pain so severe that lack of medical attention could result in the following[18]:

- Placing the patient's health in serious jeopardy
- Serious impairment to bodily functions
- Serious dysfunction of any bodily organ or part

All those eligible for Medicaid regardless of immigration status or age have access to emergency medical care so long as the above conditions are met. For these purposes, emergency medical care includes child labor and delivery.[18]

5. **How do these issues prevent an individual from becoming a "public charge"?**

Under the Immigration and Naturalization Act §212(a)(4), the Department of State and the Immigration and Naturalization Service determine whether an individual seeking admission into the United States, or seeking adjustment of status, "is likely to become a public charge" on the US government (that is, that person cannot support himself or herself and must depend on government cash benefits for an income. Such a determination would either make that person deportable or it would void his or her request for admission into the country. On May, 26, 1999, the Department of Justice issued a proposed rule to clarify the confusion and fear created by the lack of a clear standard. A person may receive benefits under Medicaid, the State Children's Health Insurance Program, and other health services without fear that doing so will affect that person's immigration status. Only when the person must rely on Medicaid for long-term care is the issue of becoming a public charge a concern. Furthermore, public benefits are specific to an individual. If a mother is applying for Medicaid for her children, she only needs to provide the children's social security number, not the social security number of the mother or anyone else in the family. Nor should the government inquire into the immigration status of anyone else in the family who is not seeking a public benefit.

6. **Do farmworker children qualify for Medicaid?**
   Children of farmworker families qualify for Medicaid so long as the above requirements for eligibility are met. Unlike the Migrant Health Act, which provided specifically for children in farmworker families, the 1996 welfare legislation bases eligibility on criteria that does not distinguish between type of labor or ages.

7. **What does Medicaid pay for?[13]**
   While each state decides what its Medicaid program will cover, the following is a list of services the state must pay for in sufficient amount, duration, and scope:

   - Inpatient hospital services
   - Outpatient hospital services
   - Physician services
   - Rural health clinic services
   - Community and migrant health clinic services
   - Preventive care and treatment for children
   - Nursing facilities services for persons age 21 or older
   - Family planning services and supplies
   - Services furnished by a licensed nurse-midwife
   - Home health services for persons entitled to receive nursing services
   - Services furnished by a certified pediatric nurse practitioner

The law also requires that the following services be covered *for children:*

- Medical care or other types of remedial care
- Private duty nursing services
- Dental services
- Physical therapy
- Prescription drugs
- Dentures
- Eyeglasses
- Prosthetic devices
- Intermediary care facility services
- Hospice care
- Services provided by a certified pediatric nurse practitioner or family nurse practitioner
- Case management services
- Community-supported independent living arrangement services
- Respiratory care services
- Tuberculosis-related services
- Personal care services
- Other diagnostic, screening, preventive, and rehabilitative services

8. What is Early and Periodic Screening, Diagnosis, and Treatment?

Medicaid covers Early and Periodic Screening, Diagnosis, and Treatment (EPSDT). The federally mandated EPSDT program was created to support the health care needs of all children under age 21 who are eligible for Medicaid; it is free of cost to participants. This program is required to provide medical, vision, hearing, and dental screening to those younger than age 21. In addition to a comprehensive physical and mental health assessment, each child is eligible for any treatment required for a physical or mental condition diagnosed during a screening.[13] Under EPSDT, children are eligible to receive treatment for all services normally covered by Medicaid.

9. What is the relationship between AFDC and TANF?

The new welfare reform law eliminates the AFDC cash benefits program and replaces it with TANF.[19] Families who met the AFDC eligibility criteria prior to welfare reform will continue to be eligible for Medicaid. The requirement that Medicaid eligibility be denied because of a loss in TANF benefits for failure to meet the work requirement specifically exempts pregnant women and children. The following individuals are eligible[16]:

- Those receiving AFDC.

- Those receiving SSI, or in states using more restrictive criteria, those aged, blind, and disabled individuals who meet criteria more restrictive than that of the SSI program.

- Infants born to Medicaid-eligible pregnant women for the first year of life.

- Children younger than age 6 and pregnant women who meet the state's AFDC financial requirements or whose family income is at or below 133% of the federal poverty level. States are required to extend Medicaid eligibility until age 19 to all children born after September 30, 1983, in families with incomes at or below the federal poverty level.

- Adoption assistance and foster care assistance recipients under Title IV-E of the Social Security Act.

- Special protected groups who lose cash assistance because of the cash programs' rules but who may be eligible for Medicaid coverage for a period of time.

Vaccines for Children

The CDC Vaccines for Children (VFC) program was begun in 1994 to immunize *all* children younger than age 2 without regard to any limitations, such as those imposed by the Welfare Reform Act. The VFC program covers the following children: (1) children receiving Medicaid, (2) uninsured children (regardless of their documentation status), (3) children whose private insurance does not cover vaccines, and (4) Native American and Alaskan Native children. The program pays for all vaccines recommended by the Advisory Committee on Immunization Practices and approved by the CDC.[13]

Special Supplemental Nutrition Program for Women, Infants, and Children (WIC)

The Special Supplemental Nutrition Program for Women, Infants, and Children (WIC) is administered by a branch of the US Department of Agriculture (USDA). This program provides a combination of nutritional supplementation, nutritional education and counseling, and increased access to health care and social service professionals for pregnant, breastfeeding, and post-partum women and infants and children up to the age of 5 years.[20] In particular, the government is interested in making the WIC program accessible to migrant and seasonal farmworkers and their children and maintains a record of the enrollment by this segment of the population in the WIC program.

1. Who is eligible for the WIC program?[20]

   • Pregnant women

   • Breastfeeding or postpartum women

   • Infants up to the age of 1 year

   • Children 1 through 4 years old

Each applicant in these categories also must be found to be (1) income eligible and (2) at nutritional risk.

2. **Are there any eligibility requirements based on immigration status?**

The states cannot deny these benefits on the basis of citizenship, alienage, or immigration status to any individual eligible to receive free public education under state or local law. At this time, no state denies free education.

Policies Regarding Foster Care, Adoption, and Children With Special Needs

The health care needs of children in foster care and children with special needs are unique, and access to health care and health insurance is crucial to them. Providing comprehensive and coordinated health care to all children in foster care is the responsibility of each state or county in its role as in loco parentis.[21] Both the state/county and the court have legal responsibility for these children even though their physical custody may be entrusted to a child welfare agency or to foster parents. Similarly, adoption assistance available from the federal, state, and county government includes access to necessary health care for all children with special needs who are adopted.[21]

This system of adoption subsidies was created to encourage the adoption of children with special needs. While adoptive parents become responsible for accessing health care for their adoptive children, adoption assistance may include a link to health care through Medicaid. This system of aid for all children in foster care and those with special needs was created under Title IV-E of the Social Security Act, and it was enacted under the Child Welfare Act in 1980.[21] To determine what steps are required to enroll migrant children and migrant children with special needs in foster care and/or adoption, it is important to contact the appropriate child welfare agency in that state.

State Children's Health Insurance Program (SCHIP)

The Balanced Budget Act of 1997 created the State Children's Health Insurance Program (SCHIP), under Title XXI of the Social Security Act, to "initiate and expand" health insurance coverage for uninsured children.[22] Federal matching funds became available for states to either expand their Medicaid programs or to create a SCHIP.[17] The federal government, through the US Department of Health and Human Services (DHHS), must approve each SCHIP plan on a state-by-state basis. Funding will be allocated according to a formula based on the number of uninsured, low-income children in each state.[22] The same limitations based on immigration status described under the Medicaid section apply to SCHIP.

Title XXI of the Social Security Act requires the states to describe the specific steps the SCHIP plan will take to target and enroll eligible low-income children. Lower income children must be covered before higher income children, and the plan may not deny eligibility to children based on a preexisting condition.[23] Each state plan must consist of one of the following: (1) the plan must be equivalent to the standard Blue Cross/Blue Shield Preferred Provider option offered to federal employees, (2) the state employee health plan, (3) the HMO with the largest commercial enrollment in the state, (4) coverage must have a value that is at least equivalent to one of the benchmark packages, (5) coverage can fall under an existing comprehensive state-based coverage, or (6) the secretary of DHHS can determine whether coverage is appropriate for targeted low-income children.[23]

States are given great flexibility to decide whether to expand Medicaid or whether to develop a separate health insurance program. Most states have, therefore, used this program to significantly increase income eligibility levels. However, most states also have included residency in the state as a requirement for eligibility. Thus, it might be necessary for each state to negotiate with other states to provide reciprocal services for children of migrant families.

School Entry

Each state has its own laws and policies regarding the age children must enter school, whether the state or school district must provide kindergarten, and whether children must attend kindergarten if it is provided. There is much variation within the states regarding compulsory school attendance age and whether kindergarten is provided with state funds. Most states do require that children start school by age 7, although a few do not require attendance until the child is 8 years old.

Children have the right to a free public education, even if they reside in a community for a short period of time. If kindergarten is provided by the state, migrant children are eligible to attend. A 1982 Supreme Court decision (*Plyer v. Doe, 457 US 202*) guarantees children the right to a free public education regardless of immigrant status. Currently, it is a violation of a child's civil rights to deny access to school based on immigration status, although some states are now challenging the constitution on this point.

There are not enough preschool programs in the country to serve all preschool children; there are even fewer that address the unique cultural and language needs of migrant preschoolers. Head Start, funded through the Administration for Children and Families (ACF) within the US Department of Health and Human Services, offers comprehensive services including health education and social services. It has provided critical leadership in bilingual/multicultural programming, parent education, and mainstreaming children with special needs. Migrant Head Start also is funded through the ACF to serve migrant children seasonally.[24] If a migrant child participated in either program in another state, there should be a medical record including immunizations, tuberculosis clearance, and other relevant information that can be obtained for school entry. Access to this information also can prevent over-immunizing children who are up to date but lack documentation.

Although a lack of records from previous schools can make it difficult for a school to identify a newly enrolled child's needs and make an appropriate placement, schools cannot legally bar a child from school. However, in the absence of proof of immunizations and tuberculosis clearance, a child's right to enter school cannot supersede the compelling public health concern for ensuring that all children are fully immunized. Schools are much better positioned to give migrant children opportunities to learn if they have access to information about the child. Health care professionals can assist families by providing copies of children's health records when they know they are leaving the area.[25]

References

1. Fair Labor Standards Act, 29 USC § 203(l) (1996) [hereinafter FLSA]
2. González M, Kurre L. *Young Agricultural Workers in California*. Berkeley, Calif: Labor Occupational Health Program, Center for Occupational and Environmental Health, School of Public Health, University of California; 1997:33-34
3. Migrant Clinicians Network. *Migrant Health Provider Orientation Manual*. Austin, Tex: Migrant Clinicians Network; 1997
4. FLSA, 29 USC §212(a)
5. FLSA, 29 USC §212(b)
6. FLSA, 29 USC §212(c)
7. DOL Seeks Help to Find Child Laborers Vol XVII series 8 *AFOP Washington Newsline*. 3 February 1998
8. Martin P. *Migrant Farmworkers and their Children*. ERIC Clearinghouse on Rural Education and Small Schools (No. ED 376 997)
9. National Advisory Council on Migrant Health. *1993 Recommendations of the National Advisory Council of Migrant Health*. Rockville, Md: National Advisory Council on Migrant Health, Bureau of Primary Health Care; 1993:17

10. Migrant Health Act, 42 USC § 254b(a)(2) (1996)

11. Id, 42 USC §254b(a)(3)

12. Id, 42 USC §254b(a)(1)(H)

13. Hershkoff H, Loffredo S. *The Rights of the Poor: The Authoritative ACLU Guide to Poor People's Rights.* Carbondale, Ill: Southern Illinois University Press; 1997

14. American Academy of Pediatrics. *Health Insurance Status of Children Under Age 19: 1999 Projections.* Elk Grove Village, Ill: American Academy of Pediatrics; 1999

15. National Health Law Program, National Center for Youth Law, National Senior Citizens Law Center. The welfare law and its effects on Medicaid recipients. *Clearinghouse Rev.* January-February 1997;1008

16. Super DA, Parrott S, Steinmetz S, Mann C. *The New Welfare Law.* [Center on Budget and Policy Priorities.] August 13, 1996. Available at: http://www.cbpp.org/ WCNSUM.HTM. Accessed February 23, 2000

17. Perkins J, Rivera L, Olson K, English A, Teare C. EPSDT Update for Child Health Insurance and Medicaid Advocates. [National Health Law Program Web site]. November 20, 1997. Available at: http://www.healthlaw.org/ pubs/child1997epsdtupdate.html. Accessed February 23, 2000

18. Health Care Financing Administration. *State Medicaid Manual 45-3: Changes Due to Welfare Reform, Part III.* Washington, DC Health Care Financing Administration; September 1997

19. Health Care Financing Administration. Medicaid welfare reform fact sheet #1: link between Medicaid and temporary assistance for needy families (TANF). Available at: http:// www.hcfa.gov/medicaid/wrfs1.htm. Accessed February 23, 2000

20. United States Department of Agriculture. WIC program and participants characteristics, April 1994 (summary). Available at: http://fns1.usda.gov/oane/MENU/Published/ WIC/files/0313.txt. Accessed February 23, 2000

21. English A, Freundlich M. Medicaid: a key to health care for foster children and adopted children with special needs Vol 31 series 3-4 clearinghouse review. *J Poverty Law.* 110 (July-August 1997)

22. Health Care Financing Administration. Children's Health Insurance Program, Letter to State Officials (August 27, 1997)

23. Balanced Budget Act of 1997, Public Law 105-33, Title IV: Medicare, Medicaid, and Children's Health Provisions: State Children's Health Insurance Program, Subtitle J, §2102. Available at: http://www.migrantclinicians.org. Accessed: February 23, 2000

24. Migrant Head Start. Report. 1989

25. National Association for the Education of Young Children. *Good Teaching Practices for Older Preschoolers and Kindergartners: A Position Statement of the National Association for the Education of Young Children.* Washington, DC: National Association for the Education of Young Children. 1990

Resources

American Academy of Pediatrics
141 Northwest Point Blvd
Elk Grove Village, IL 60007
Telephone: 847/434-4000
Web site: http://www.aap.org

Migrant Clinicians Network, Inc.
PO Box 164285
Austin, TX 78716
Telephone: 512/327-2017
Fax: 512/327-0719
E-mail: mcn@onr.com
Web site: http://www.migrantclinician.org

Vaccines for Children
Web site: http://www.cdc.gov/nip/vfc/
Each state and region has a designated VFC coordinator.
For more infomration, visit the Web site or call the CDC
National Immunization Information Hotline: 800/232-2522.

Index

A

Abdomen examination, well-child
    visits and, 48
Acquired immunodeficiency
    syndrome (AIDS), 113
Acute poisoning
    diagnosis and treatment of, 91
    through lead, 84–85
    through pesticides, 89–90
Adolescent care
    health promotion for, 64
    obtaining history for, 62–63
    overview of, 62
    physical examination for, 63–64
    special considerations for, 65–66
Adoption of children, policies
    regarding, 173
Agricultural injuries. *See* Injuries
Agricultural workers. *See* Migrant
    farmworkers
Aid to Families with Dependent
    Children (AFDC), 164, 171
Aliens, Medicaid benefits to, 166
American Academy of Pediatrics, 153
American Cancer Society, 154
American College of Obstetricians
    and Gynecologists, 154
American Heart Association, 154
American Social Health Association,
    154
AmeriSpan Unlimited, 150
Anemia
    hypochromic microcytic, 85
    iron-deficiency, 80
Animal-related injuries, 100

B

Balanced Budget Act, 163, 165, 174
BCG vaccine, 55, 110
Bilingual interpreter. *See* Interpreter(s)
Binational Migrant Education
    Program, 36
Boston Language Institute, The, 150,
    160
Bottle feeding
    vs breastfeeding, 11
    early childhood caries and, 14, 70
    oral health and, 72
Breastfeeding
    early weaning of, 76
    issues for migrant women, 11–12
    oral health and, 72
    ways to encourage, 13
Brujos, 23

C

Caída de la mollera (sunken fontanel),
    18
Carbamate poisoning
    diagnosis and treatment of, 91
    symptoms of, 90
Cardiovascular examination,
    well-child visits and, 47
Caries
    early childhood, 14, 69–70
    from hypoplasia, 69
    occlusal, 69
    patterns, 70
    preventive treatments for, 70,
    73–74
    smooth surface, 69

Cariogenic bacteria, oral health and, 68
Caustic alkali, 101
CDC Vaccines for Children (VFC) program, 172
Ceramics, lead poisoning through imported, 84
Chagas' disease
    clinical manifestations of, 112
    prevalence of, 111–112
Chelation therapy, treating lead poisoning with, 87, 88
Chemicals. *See* Pesticides
Child abuse
    assessing family problems related to, 97–98
    cupping treatment confused with, 22
    discipline issues and, 15
    interventions for treating, 98
    overview of, 96
Child labor laws, 104, 161
Children. *See also* Migrant children
    discipline practices used for, 15–16
    Hispanic families' views about development of, 16
    policies regarding age for school entry for, 175–176
    with special needs, policies regarding, 173
    susceptibility to pesticide poisoning, 88
Child Welfare Act, 173
Citizenship, Medicaid eligibility requirements and, 165–166
Clinicians. *See* Health care professionals

Communication
    with bilingual interpreters, 31–32, 65
    ways to improve, with farmworkers, 8
Comprehensive care, ways to improve, 26
Congenital syphilis, 114
Consecutive interpretation, defined, 33
Contaminated dust and soil, lead poisoning through, 84
Conversation and phrase books for medical personnel, 148–149
Crew leaders' role in treatment plans, 10
Cross-cultural medicine
    concept of, 6–7
    overcoming language barriers in, 7
    practicing within social context and, 24
    ways to improve communication in, 8
Culture-bound syndromes, 17, 18
Cupping treatment, 22
Curanderos, 23
Cutaneous leishmaniasis, 112–113

D

Dental caries. *See* Caries
Dental diseases. *See also* Oral health
    assessment of, 71
    patterns in, 68–70
    preventive treatments for fighting, 73–75
Denver Development test, 44
Dependents. *See* Migrant children
Diccionario de Especialidades, 24
Dietary habits. *See* Nutritional status
Dimercaptosuccinic Acid (DMSA), 87

Distance learning program in Mexico, 35
Drinking water, lead poisoning through, 84

E

Ear examination, well-child visits and, 46–47
Early and Periodic Screening, Diagnosis, and Treatment (EPSDT) program, 170, 171
Early childhood caries, 14
in migrant children, 67, 69
prevention of, 70
Early developmental delays, lead poisoning and, 85
Education
mobility patterns impact on children's, 51–52
parents' role in children's, 52–54
Educational systems
in Mexico, 34–36
US vs Mexico, 35t
Empacho, 18
Empirical therapy, 25
Enamel, demineralized, identification of, 71
Encephalopathy, lead poisoning and, 84–85, 87
Environmental concerns
groundwater contamination, 94–95
lead poisoning, 83–88
pesticide poisoning, 88–94
Equipment related injuries, 100, 102–103
Evil eye, 18
Explanatory model approach, 19–21
Eye examination, well-child visits and, 47

F

Fair Labor Standards Act (FLSA), 161–162
Falls, injuries associated with, 101
Family members as interpreters, 31
Farming
injuries associated with, 102–103
pesticide poisoning and, 88–94
Farmworker Health Services, Inc, 139
Farmworker Justice Fund, Inc, 139
Farmworkers. See Migrant farmworkers
Financial barriers to health care, 24–25
Fluoride supplements/varnish
preventing dental decay with, 73–75
protocols for prescribing, 74t
Folk health care practices, 22–23
Folk medicines, lead poisoning through, 84
Food, used as a reward by Hispanic families, 14
Foster care, policies regarding, 173
Frequent moves. See Mobility patterns

G

Genitalia and Tanner Staging, well-child visits and, 48
Ghost Ranch Conference Center, 151
Gingivae, oral health and, 73
Global Exchange, 151, 160
Groundwater contamination
intestinal parasitic infestation related to, 110–111
nitrate contamination related to, 95
overview of, 94–95
recommendations for handling, 95

Growth and development assessment
    common findings in, 49
    Denver Development test for,
        44–46

H

Hansen's disease, 115
Health care
    adapting, to lifestyle of migrant
        children, 27
    financial barriers to, 24–25
    in Mexico, 23–24
    needs of children in foster care,
        173
Health care professionals
    breastfeeding issues and, 11–12
    continuity with, 26
    conversation and phrase books
        for, 148–149
    cross-cultural medicine concept
        for, 6–7
    handling parenting beliefs issues
        and, 11
    language resources for, 147–149
    recommendations for adolescent
        care by, 65–66
    recommendations for groundwater
        contamination by, 94–95
    recommendations for immuniza-
        tions by, 61
    recommendations for improving
        dietary habits by, 80–82
    recommendations for injury pre-
        vention by, 106–107
    recommendations for oral health
        by, 71
    recommendations for pesticide
        poisoning by, 93
    recommendations for well-child
        visits by, 50

    use of interpreters by, 29–30
    ways to improve communication
        with farmworkers by, 8
Health promotion materials in
        Spanish, sources for, 153–158
Healthy Mothers, Healthy Babies
        Coalition, 154
Herbal teas used in home remedies,
        22
Hispanic families
    discussing taboo subjects with,
        7–8
    folk health care practices used
        by, 22–23
    health belief models of, 16–17
    healthy baby concept of, 14
    infant feeding practices used
        by, 13–15
    labor force, 3
    self-care treatments used by,
        21–22
HIV infection, 113–114
Home remedies
    lead poisoning through, 84
    used by Hispanic families, 21–22
Hypochromic microcytic anemia, 85
Hypoplasia, caries from, 69

I

Immigration and Naturalization
        Act, 168
Immigration status
    of migrant children, 3–4
    public education and, 175
Immunizations
    barriers to age-appropriate, 57
    linking physical examination
        and, 57, 61
    obtaining history for, 55–56
    overview of, 55

policies regarding school entry and, 175–176
treatment plans for obtaining, 61
Infant feeding
bottle feeding and, 11, 14, 70, 72
breastfeeding and, 11–12, 13, 72, 76
practices used by Hispanic mothers, 13–15
Infectious diseases
congenital syphilis, 114–115
human immunodeficiency virus infection, 113–114
intestinal parasitic infestation, 110–111
leishmaniasis, 112–113
leprosy, 115
malaria, 113
overview of, 108
tissue protozoan infections, 111–112
tuberculosis, 108–110
Injuries
data on, 99–100
overview of, 99
risk factors for developing, 101–104
types of, 100–101
ways to control, 104, 105–106, 107
Intensive learning programs
AmeriSpan Unlimited, 150
Boston Language Institute, The, 150, 160
Ghost Ranch Conference Center, 151
Global Exchange, 151, 160
Spanish Abroad, Inc, 152
Studyabroad.com, 152
Internet, learning on, 152

Interpreter(s)
bilingual, 28
certified, 28, 29
family member/friend as, 31
how to find, 32
need to use, 31–32
qualifications for, 30
recommendations for working with, 33
role in adolescent care, 65
services, telephone, 32
trained, 29–30
unqualified, 31
Intestinal parasitic infestation
clinical manifestations of, 111
overview of, 110–111
IQ scores, lead poisoning and lower, 85
Iron-deficiency anemia, 80

K

Kala-azar, 113

L

Laboratory screenings for well-child visits, 50
Labor force, Hispanic, 3
Language barriers
in cross-cultural medicine, 7
interpreters for handling, 29–30
of migrant farmworkers, 3–4, 28–29
to oral health, 67
Language resources
conversation and phrase books for medical personnel, 148–149
for learning Haitian Creole language, 158–160
medical dictionary, 147
self-study guides, 147–148

Laws
    related to child abuse, 96, 97
    related to child labor, 104, 161
    related to foster care and adoption
        issues, 173
Lead poisoning
    effects of, 84–86
    evaluating children for, 86
    guidelines for diagnosing, 86–88
    overview of, 83
    sources of, 83–84
Leishmaniasis
    clinical manifestations of, 112–113
    incubation period for, 112
Leprosy, 115
Lower-dose exposure to lead, effects
    of, 85

M

Machinery related injuries, 100,
    102–103
Malaria, 113
Mal de ojo (evil eye), 18
Mantoux tuberculin skin test, 109
Measles vaccine, 56
Medicaid benefits, 24, 25, 67
    AFDC and TANF programs and,
        171
    to aliens, 166
    citizenship status and, 165–166
    eligibility requirements for,
        164–165, 167t
    EPSDT program and, 170–171
    to non-qualified aliens, 166, 168
    overview of, 163
    "public charge" issues under,
        168–169
    SCHIP program and, 174
    services covered under, 169–170

Medical jargon, cross-cultural
    medicine concept and, 6–7
Mental health issues, migrant
    farmworkers and, 63
Methemoglobinemia, symptoms
    of, 95t
Mexican immunization schedule, 56t
Mexico
    educational systems in, 34–36
    health care in, 23–24
    obtaining prescription drugs in,
        21, 24
Migrant adolescents
    acculturation in, 66
    injuries among, 99, 100, 102
    screening recommendations for,
        63–65
    teenage pregnancy in, 63
Migrant children
    abuse of, 96–98
    adolescent care of, 62–66
    CDC Vaccines for Children (VFC)
        program for, 172
    discipline practices used for,
        15–16
    early childhood caries in, 14, 67,
        69–70
    EPSDT program for, 170–171
    groundwater contamination
        among, 94–95
    growth and development assess-
        ment findings in, 49
    Head Start programs for, 141–142,
        175
    immigration status of, 3–4
    immunizations for, 55–57, 58t, 60t
    infectious diseases in, 108–115
    injuries among, 99–107
    language barriers of, 3–4
    lead poisoning among, 83–88
    Medicaid eligibility requirements
        for, 164–165, 167t, 169

mobility patterns of, 2, 3
nutritional status of, 76–82
obesity among, 14–15
oral health of, 67–75
pesticide poisoning among, 88–94
SCHIP program for, 174
school readiness issues of, 51–54
ways to adapt health care to
   lifestyle of, 27
well-child visits of, 43–48
Migrant Clinicians Network, Inc, 140
Migrant Education Program, 140–141
Migrant families
   child discipline practices used by,
      15–16
   ways to encourage breastfeeding
      in, 13
Migrant farmworkers. *See also*
   Hispanic families
   cross-cultural medicine concept
      and, 6–8
   defined, 1
   explanatory model approach used
      by, 19–21
   Fair Labor Standards Act and,
      161–162
   family structure of, 9–10
   federal programs for, 4–5
   financial barriers to health care
      for, 24–25
   health belief models of, 6, 9,
      16–17
   history of, 1
   HIV infection among, 113–114
   incidence of TB among, 108–110
   intestinal parasitic infestation
      among, 110–111
   language barriers of, 3–4, 28–29
   leishmaniasis among, 112–113

leprosy among, 115
living conditions of, 4, 68
malaria among, 113
Medicaid eligibility requirements
   for, 164–165, 167t
mental health issues of, 63
Migrant Health Programs for, 142,
   162–163
mobility patterns of, 2, 3, 51–52,
   57
nomadic, 2
point-to-point, 2
programs and organizations related
   to, 139–146
sexually transmitted diseases
   among, 114
states with largest population of, 2t
tissue protozoan infections among,
   111–112
transportation problems of, 25
Migrant Head Start, 141–142, 175
Migrant Health Program, 1, 142,
   162–163
Migrant Health Promotion, 142–143,
   155
Migrant women
   breastfeeding issues for, 11–12
   infant feeding practices used by,
      13–15
   teenage pregnancy in, 63
Mind-body dichotomy notion, 6
Mobility patterns
   impact on children's education,
      51–52
   impact on children's immuniza-
      tions, 57
   impact on health care needs, 26
   of migrant farmworkers, 2, 3
Mucosal leishmaniasis, 113

N

National Advisory Council on
Migrant Health, 143
National Agriculture Workers Survey
(NAWS), 1
National AIDS Clearinghouse, 155
National Alliance for Hispanic
Health, 156
National Association of Community
Health Centers, Inc, 144
National Cancer Institute, 155
National Center for Farmworker
Health, Inc, 144
National Clearinghouse for Alcohol
and Drug Information, 155
National Diabetes Information
Clearinghouse, 156
National Digestive Disease
Information Clearinghouse,
156
National Immigration Law Center,
144–145
National Institute for Occupational
Safety and Health, 157
National Institute of Mental
Health, 157
National Institutes of Health, 156
National Lead Safety Council, 157
National Rural Health Association,
145
National Safety Council, 157
Neglect. See Child abuse
Nervous system, lead poisoning and
impairment to, 85
Neurologic screening, well-child visits
and, 48
N-methyl carbamate poisoning
diagnosis and treatment of, 91
symptoms of, 90

Non-qualified aliens, Medicaid
benefits to, 168
Nutritional status
laboratory screenings for
assessing, 80
obtaining history for assessing,
77–78
overview of, 76
physical examination for
assessing, 78–80
recommendations for improving,
80–82

O

Obesity, prevalence of, 14–15, 78–80
Occlusal caries, 69
Occupational Safety and Health
Administration (OSHA), 103
Oral health
assessment for disease prevention
and, 71
barriers to, 67–68
dental diseases patterns and,
68–70
dental examination and, 70–71
overview of, 67
promotion and education, 72–73
Organophosphate poisoning
diagnosis and treatment of, 91
symptoms of, 90

P

Paraquat, exposure to, 91
Parents' role in stimulating learning
in children, 52–54
PBS Adult Learning Service, 152
Personal Responsibility and Work
Opportunity Reconciliation
Act of 1996, 164, 165

Pesticide poisoning
    children susceptibility to, 88
    diagnosis of, 89–91
    management of, 92
    overview of, 88–89
    preventive counseling for, 93–94
Pesticides
    injuries associated with, 101
    practices, avoiding unsafe, 93
    practices, using safe, 93–94
    routes of exposure to, 89
Physical examination
    for adolescent care, 63–64
    for assessing nutritional status,
        78–80
    dental examination as part of,
        70–71
    immunizations and, 57, 61
    for school readiness, 52
    screening recommendations for, 65
    for well-child visits, 46–48
Plasmodium infection, 113
Poisoning
    lead, 83–88
    pesticide, 88–94
Pottery, lead poisoning through
    imported, 84
Poverty
    child abuse and, 98
    impact on children's education, 51
    migrant farmworkers and, 4
Premenstrual syndrome, 17
Prenatal health care
    congenital syphilis and, 114
    oral health as part of, 72–73
Prescription drugs in Mexico, 21, 24
Public clinics in Mexico, 23
Public education
    barriers to, 34
    immigration status and, 175
    in Mexico, 34–35

Pulmonary examination, well-child
    visits and, 47

R

Remote-simultaneous interpretation
    service, 32
Rollover protection structures
    (ROPS), 102
Rural Community Assistance
    Program, 145–146

S

Safe Drinking Water Act, 94
School readiness
    obtaining family's history for,
        51–52
    overview of, 51
    physical examination for, 52
    stimulating learning in children
        and, 52–54
Self-care treatments used by Hispanic
    farmworkers, 21–22
Self-study guides, 147–148, 159
Sexually transmitted diseases,
    114–115
Simultaneous interpretation, defined,
    33
Skin examination, well-child visits
    and, 46
Smooth surface caries, 69
Sobadores, 23
Social Security Act, 171, 173, 174
Spanish Abroad, Inc, 152
Special Supplemental Nutrition
    Program for Women, Infants,
    and Children (WIC), 172–173
State Children's Health Insurance
    Program (SCHIP), 174
Strepmutans bacteria, 69
Study abroad programs, 150–152, 160

Substance Abuse and Mental Health
  Services Administration, 153
Summary interpretation, defined, 33
Sunken fontanel, 18
Supplemental Security Income (SSI),
  164, 165, 166
Susto, 18
Syphilis, congenital, 114–115

T

Tecla (Internet learning source), 152
Teenage pregnancy, 63
Telephone(s)
  interpreter services, 32
  problems of migrant farmworkers,
    25
Temporary Assistance for Needy
  Families (TANF), 166, 171
Texas Department of Health, 158
Tissue protozoan infections
  clinical manifestations of, 112
  prevalence of, 111–112
Tooth decay
  in migrant children, 68–69
  recognizing, 70
  ways to prevent, 72–75
Translator. *See* Interpreter(s)
Transportation problems of migrant
  farmworkers, 25
Treatment plans
  crew leaders' role in, 10
  migrants' family structure impact
    on, 9–10

for obtaining immunizations, 61
using explanatory model approach
  for, 19–21
ways to improve communication
  of, 8
Trypanosomiasis, 111–112
Tuberculosis
  clinical manifestations of, 109
  diagnosis of, 109–110
  incidence of, 108
  management of patients with, 110

V

Viceral leishmaniasis, 113
Violence, injuries associated with, 101

W

Welfare Reform Act, 172
Well-child visits
  assessment and health care plan
    and, 50
  laboratory screenings for, 50
  obtaining medical history for,
    44–46
  overview of, 43
  physical examination for, 46–48
  registration for, 43
WIC, 172–173

X

Xylitol gum, preventing dental decay
  with, 75